Face Reading

Discover How to Read People Like Clockwork

(Self-care and Natural Healing Through Traditional Chinese Medicine)

Michael Snider

Published By **Regina Loviusher**

Michael Snider

All Rights Reserved

Face Reading: Discover How to Read People Like Clockwork (Self-care and Natural Healing Through Traditional Chinese Medicine)

ISBN 978-1-77485-495-2

No part of this guidebook shall be reproduced in any form without permission in writing from the publisher except in the case of brief quotations embodied in critical articles or reviews.

Legal & Disclaimer

The information contained in this ebook is not designed to replace or take the place of any form of medicine or professional medical advice. The information in this ebook has been provided for educational & entertainment purposes only.

The information contained in this book has been compiled from sources deemed reliable, and it is accurate to the best of the Author's knowledge; however, the Author cannot guarantee its accuracy and validity and cannot be held liable for any errors or omissions. Changes are periodically made to this book. You must consult your doctor or get professional medical advice before using any of the suggested remedies, techniques, or information in this book.

Upon using the information contained in this book, you agree to hold harmless the

Author from and against any damages, costs, and expenses, including any legal fees potentially resulting from the application of any of the information provided by this guide. This disclaimer applies to any damages or injury caused by the use and application, whether directly or indirectly, of any advice or information presented, whether for breach of contract, tort, negligence, personal injury, criminal intent, or under any other cause of action.

You agree to accept all risks of using the information presented inside this book. You need to consult a professional medical practitioner in order to ensure you are both able and healthy enough to participate in this program.

TABLE OF CONTENTS

INTRODUCTION 1

CHAPTER 1: BASIC FORM OF FACE AND HEAD 5

CHAPTER 2: EYES AND EYEBROWS 12

CHAPTER 3: NOW TO THE EYE ITSELF 15

CHAPTER 4: NOW TO THE MOUTH" THAT'S ALSO VERY IMPORTANT. 23

CHAPTER 5: WHAT IS CHINESE FACE READING? 25

CHAPTER 6: WHAT DO CHINESE FACE READING DETERMINE ILLNESS WITHIN THE BODY? 30

CHAPTER 7: FACE READING 49

CHAPTER 8: ANALYSIS OF DECEPTION AND YOU 65

CHAPTER 9: LEARN MORE DETAILS ABOUT YOUR AMAZING FOREHEAD 73

CHAPTER 10: FEAR IS IT'S HARD TO CREATE 81

CHAPTER 11: ARE YOU JUST DISGUSTED, OR A PSYCHOPATH? 88

CHAPTER 12: THE TWO BIG MYTHS OF DECEPTION ANALYSIS 94

CHAPTER 13: HOW TO LEARN THE SIX UNIVERSAL EMOTIONS 100

CHAPTER 14: WHAT IS IT MEAN WHEN A GIRL OR SOMEONE SAYS "SURPRISE" ME? 106

CHAPTER 15: WHAT DOES ONE MANAGE THEIR ANGER? 112

CHAPTER 16: A FEW COMBINATION FACE EXPRESSIONS 116

CHAPTER 17: PARTITION OF TWO SECTIONS OF THE FACE 126

CHAPTER 18: EIGHTEEN MOST IMPORTANT FACTS ABOUT YOUR FACE 134

CHAPTER 19: CATEGORY THE FACE IN ITS WIDTH 143

CONCLUSION 184

Introduction

She was an avid Scouser and had created an investigation of the faces she read. She studied the shape lines, length, width as well as the eyebrows' shape, lips, eyes, and so and on.

She believed she could determine the character of anyone by simply just looking at them.

I didn't believe any of it until I got engaged to my potential partner (her daughter) and she accompanied us to visit my family members - mother as well as father and my older sister.

Everyone was on top of their game manners and polite, and the meeting was smooth with everyone acting perfectly.

But a few months later, following the wedding my mother-in-law was in town for a couple of days after having returned from Liverpool.

While we sat down to the tea she mentioned that she was able to seen my family's faces, and then she shared the whole story of their personalities which were not displayed during the polite meeting.

My mother-in-law was absolutely right. She claimed that my father was an uncontrollable and violent temper, yet was a clever.

She told me that my sister was artistic, and she was - an artist of the highest caliber however, she was also a bit snarky and a liar. This is also true.

She told me that my mother was smart - as a teacher at school - and gentle, but she was also a bit intolerant of contradictions - which is the truth.

All of this was not displayed the first time my mother-in-law met with my family however, she had told me about their stories like she'd known them for a long time.

Of course, what she said to my fiancée (her daughter) about me, based on her studying my face I don't know however the wedding went forward.

My mother-in-law passed away some time ago, but throughout my time with her, she was always talking about people she were watching - often on television or on television "God is a fan of the tone of his voice. Just take a look at how long his neck and the man will never stop talking."

Perhaps she'd look at a photograph in the paper - "He's a clever guy however, he's as hard as nails. There's no point crying on his shoulder and expressing your woes. You won't find any sympathy from him."

She could also talk about a neighbor who recently moved into the next house: "God! She's neurotic. Beware of her!"

It's true that I'm very elderly (85) and won't remain here for long. However, my son is saying that he'd like to be in a position to read people's faces just as his Grandma in Law used to do.

So I'm noting down the things I remember from the things my mother-in-law in law had to say about face reading throughout the years I spent with her.

I have never found her to be in error as I gained more information about the person who was at issue.

Of course, we have to be aware that both women and men have a lot more "beauty" treatment than they did back in the earlier days.

A lot of individuals have eyebrows pulled with longer and thicker eyelashes that are stuck to the lines that are removed with botox. Some also are treated with facelifts.

Some wear wigs or hair pieces, which alter or covering the height or the width of their foreheads, one of the most important factors.

You'll have to test to discern the truth and discredit it.

There is no way to make it easy is it?

Here's the details (according to me and my Scouser mother-in-law) about how to recognize character by their face.

Chapter 1: Basic Form Of Face and Head

The forehead is significant. The wider the distance between the eyebrows and hairline, the more space there is for the brain. (of course , you must ignore baldness and wigs as well as hairpieces.

If you know a person who has gone bald , you will typically see through the texture of his skin where the hairline was and you'll be able to observe the space for the brain.

Higher the height of forehead, the bigger the brain size and the smarter and more knowledgeable the person will be . On the other hand, the smaller the forehead, the smaller the brain, and consequently the less intelligent a person is.

But there's something more than this.

The forehead's width is vitally important.

If someone is tall and is straight up, not turning to the sides - they could be extremely smart, but will not think outside of the box, according to people who are trendy are known to say.

The types with narrow foreheads can get a top diploma in writing a work on Chaucer's works. Chaucer (or any other work, according to chatterboxes) making sure that every word and every refence right and reviewing all widely accepted opinions, putting these in order according to their merit and the like.

However, this straight-up forehead type is not likely to be able to come up with a fresh perspective or a fresh perspective or think of any other writer that isn't well-known who deserves to be talked about.

To think fresh on new topics or fresh ideas on subjects that you have previously thought of, you require the width of your forehead and also the height.

A person who doesn't have an imposing forehead, but rather an elongated one can make a more effective candidate for a politician, or P.R. man, because even though he may not be the most brilliantly intelligent but he'd have fresh ideas and would be able to find new ground.

If you do view reconstructions of the heads and faces of the primitive man, not necessarily homo sapiens, like us but other parts of our human tree you'll notice that a lot of them have extremely foreheads and narrow faces - and they were dead!

Brains are the only way to stay alive in the world today.

In addition, I was quite surprised to discover the other time that the stopping of being chimps , and developing tall legs, walking straight and having a modern human body shape came before creating the brain with the largest size.

There was a specific species of man known as Homo Erectus who resembled us. He walked out of the trees and stood up straight and carried tools. They spread throughout the globe and lasted for thousands and millions of years before dying out, but he had a tiny brain and a narrow, low forehead.

You might think that you need to develop a huge brain to appreciate the benefits of falling from trees, but apparently not.

Sorry to continue chatting however, I thought this little bit of information was very interesting.

How do I get back to reading faces and heads:

My mother-in-law always would say that having a moderately (not extremely) high forehead on an oval head was the mark of a successful businessman.

The person with a long brain even with a large brain, would not do very well with people in the world.

Now let's look at foreheads. Whatever shape they take their shape, the lines they form are crucial.

Naturally, lines will develop as you age but you are not able to make use of lines to read faces of young people.

A few lines, just above the nose, run both ways, while other lines that cover the majority of the forehead stretch between sides.

The upward and downward lines over the nostrils are significant.

If one person has a line running through the space, he will be extremely adept at focusing on a particular task.

The more extensive and long this line is, the more careful and focused this person is. Whatever job they are assigned, they will perform it with a fervent dedication to every aspect, with nothing being overlooked or leaving to chance.

This is the type of person who should be the main cashier in an extremely complex organization.

The disadvantage of this precision is that the more detailed and longer the line the more a person believes that the person (or they) is 100% right and that their way of doing things is the only and only way to do it, and that anyone not doing things the way they do is wrong.

Often, these individuals are correct and right in every aspect, but they can be difficult to be around when you explore a different way of doing things silly, stupid you!

If you do have this type of thought but not completely you'll be able to be able to concentrate and think with precision and will not stutter or insist that you are the only one who is correct.

Two lines running both ways on each side of this space above the nose indicate that you will be able to focus on a task and finish it with ease, however you aren't going to be precise in every aspect and doingt every I.

It is not your intention to assert that you have the best method to do things and that only you're right. You'll do your best to complete the task and accept that others may come up with better methods to accomplish it.

Based on how long or deep lines they have, it shows how solid these features are. The two line individuals are likely to be the most easy to work with for general work.

As I've mentioned, if your goal is an accountant or an organizer for a complex and important job, choose the person who has one clear line.

Have you noticed that a lot of people who are like chancellors of the exchequer are wearing that long line of hair above their noses?

Then we get to the long lines that run vertically along the front of your face. Sometimes, they are straight and only one line. Sometimes, they are split into smaller lengths.

My mother-in-law told me that people who have a single uninterrupted line will be able to follow a project from beginning to conclusion while those who has broken lines will get bored easily and move from one thing to the next.

I've been unable to determine if this is accurate or not.

Chapter 2: Eyes and Eyebrows

Eyebrows are a must However, today, eyebrows can be pulled out off, completely removed and redrawn in with makeup pencils and are generally changed so to the point that looking them may be ineffective.

If you do detect natural eyebrows, this is what you need to look for.

The more hairy and bushier they get more ferocious is the temperament of the individual.

The swollen eyebrows that meet in the middle just across the nose are an indication of an explosive and inexplicably violent temper.

Beware.

However , if the person has relatively smooth eyebrows, it is important to look at the the shape and placement.

If the eyebrows are just curving over the eyes, then that person is probably normal in their temperament.

If the ends of the nose are upwards and upwards, then the person may be prone to being skeptical.

Then look at the eyelid:

It's a little difficult to communicate however I've done my best.

If the eyelid isn't evident at all however the skin fold over the eye, which is pressed downwards by the eyebrow completely covers the eyelid (seen in a lot of politicians) This indicates that the individual is determined in achieving their goals.

There will be no turning off the idea of continuing with their personal tasks to enjoy a stunning sunset or to in search of beautiful pieces of art or to listen to some music. The job has to be completed and their goals accomplished.

Of course, this could be an advantage - it is contingent on the individual is trying to accomplish.

If you are able to see the eyelid's curvature clearly, it indicates that the individual has time for things other than reaching their goals.

One could be able to stop and admire the beautiful sky, or even take some time for a little of art as a pastime or practice piano and join your family members to sing Christmas carols around Christmas or simply to talk with friends or family members.

Of course, the eyelid covered individuals could do the same things if they were advancing the achievement of their goals.

Another thing to note while you are at this part that is the facial.

People who have a line on the nostril where spectacles rest - but that are not caused by spectacles, are likely towards selfishness.

I haven't looked into this issue much however, that's what my mother-in-law told me and who can inform the Scouser that she's wrong I certainly won't.

Chapter 3: Now To The Eye Itself

If the eye isn't big, the person is sluggish and very stingy in dealing with money.

The same person can also be amusing and humorous. I've seen these tiny eyes of a mean person in well popular comedians. Don't let their enthusiasm fool you. They're sly and serious people will remain.

One last point regarding the eye that is the eye itself. I have observed that this is indeed the case.

If the eye's white is visible throughout the colored iris (and this is quite unusual) it is an indication that you are hyperactive. If you have a partner who is like this, they'll drive you mad with their endless complaining about this and this, even though there's no reason to bother to bother them at all.

Oh, and I've completely not thought of Close Set Eyes

Close-set eyes happen when the distance between the eyes appears smaller than normal.

That means you can and should remain in the privacy of your thoughts. There's no leaking of personal information that could cause an elicitation of curiosity or even a smile.

A person is capable of keeping information and thoughts to him or her.

There are many instances of close eyes in successful criminals . This is not because they are an indication of criminality However, if you've criminal tendencies, and you keep secrets, it is the recipe to succeed in the criminal world.

If you're with someone with a couple of eye contact, you might be having a great or fun-loving time, however, you'll likely find that you're the one to get to the bar for your next batch of drinks . And perhaps after you've returned home, all your valuables could be missing - due to the fact that your charming chum has told his criminal gang they would see you out in the evening.

Noses

The Nose is so important and is so crucial.

Size of nose reveals how big the persona.

A well-crafted forehead with strong lines won't be useful when you've got a small nose. There is no way to be able to show enough character to take you far.

Noses can be found in various shapes , and all have different things. Take a look at my

A large nose with an outward-facing curve indicates an extremely large and aggressive personality. If it's also accompanied by big eyes and a wrinkle on the forehead I would advise you to get a seat on the couch.

The Duke of Wellington (Arthur Wellesley the one who won every battle) had a large nose however, it was delicately designed and had a thin boney ridge on the top of the face close to the eyes.

This signified (as Napoleon found out) that Wellington had a very likable personality, however he also had an appreciation for the arts, and could be easily offended.

If you happen to meet someone who has that bony ridge on the upper portion of their nose, you must be cautious about when you speak to them about personal comments. The offender can easily be punished.

Arthur Wellesley was a very fascinating person, and his facial features are worthy of study. Take a look and learn many things from any photo you view of his.

He certainly was one who thought outside the box.

He was well-trained in battle tactics of the day, and also was a combat veteran in India.

He returned to Europe.

In the past, in Europe there were also conventional methods of fighting battles, such as organizing your troops in a traditional manner on a predetermined field and putting the regiments in a predetermined arrangement.

Arthur Wellesley did not do this.

He'd sometimes hide an entire army under the hill's brow and then pulled it up in a flash and then sent it to battle opposing regiments in the wrong regiment's order. Of course, he always prevailed.

Commanders of the enemy were known to complain that Wellesley was not adhering to the rules.

He said he had did not feel any obligation to engage in an opponent "fairly".

The soldiers who served under Wellesley did not revere the man (he described his normal soldiers as scum from the earth) and, in contrast, sailors fighting alongside Nelson and Sir Francis Drake, who would follow their commanders into The Gates of Hell - no questions requested.

The soldiers were informed that Wellesley was going to be placed on their payroll They did not scream with excitement. They let out a sigh of relief.

Arthur Wellesley was efficient.

They knew that if Arthur was in charge, the ammunition arriving would be of the proper size for their guns. There would always be the correct amount of food , equipment, as well as tents and accommodations. Arthur was prepared.

He also didn't enjoy combat or the horrible killing.

He was not a glamour hunter like Napoleon.

Wellesley was only a fighter when it was required to accomplish his objectives. Why kill even your enemies when you didn't have to? They were also human.

Wellesley and Napoleon provide interesting contrasts.

Napoleon was the son of Revolution and Equality and down with the aristocrats.

Arther Wellesley was an aristocrat with snobbery who was elevated due to the influence of and string pulling by his great-grandparents.

Following the victory at Waterloo, Napoleon the Man of the People was forced to leave all his soldiers and raced through the countryside in a comfortable coach , and four horses to save his life and his future.

Arthur Wellesley, the son of privilege, was a frequent visitor to the battlefield, doing everything possible to get help to the wounded. When he was exhausted when he returned to his home He laid on the floor after donating his bed to wounded and dying officer.

However, to return to Noses:

A big nose indicates an impressive sign of a persona. A thin bony ridge on one end of the face indicates an passion for the arts as well as one who is easily offended.

A deflated end of the nose suggests a desire to money. A nose that's pointed and pushing forward is a curious 'nosy-parker' kind of person. A wide nose at the nostrils may suggest a tendency to be rough.

Chapter 4: Now To The Mouth" That's also very important.

Then first, the lip. My mother-in-law said that a long lip indicates an opinionated view of their personal position. I don't think I've ever had the chance to observe this in detail but you will observe this long upper lip on people who are seeking fame and attention.

Now , the mouth itself. The shape and thickness of lips show how much affection and feeling is there.

Lips of some people are so thin that they're not even visible. This is a sign of hardness of heart and no affection towards their own families. They're really as members of the "Turn your grandmother to the winter" brigade.

When lips turn slightly softer and more full They are able to feel sympathy and affection for their loved ones.

Normally, full lips are a sign of an individual who feels for their family and other people of a normal household.

You can tell them about your problems and receive empathy and perhaps some help.

A few people have a shorter, lifted-up upper lip. These individuals are loud and often utter their thoughts in a tactless manner when they are not in the mood.

I've seen it happen in politicians who are just emerging who suddenly find themselves in hot water because they say something right at the wrong moment.

Lips that are very, very full can be the sign of too emotional.

Chapter 5: What is Chinese face reading?

The History

Chinese Face reading, also referred to by the name of "Mien Shiang" is 3000 years old, and first appeared in the 6th century B.C. Face reading is a way to reveal the personality, health as well as the character of any race or culture. The practice of face reading was first discovered during the Taoist and Daoism time period, in the time of Taoist monks utilized face reading to convey information about people to the Emperor. It was highly regarded as reliable. Chinese face reading was employed as a tool for diagnosing to identify the health status and the future diseases and illnesses of individuals. Around 2600 B.C. the Yellow Emperor's classic study of Internal Medicine recorded the art of observing the exterior of the body to reveal the health state of the internal body, referring with Chinese facial reading. An in-depth understanding of TCM was beneficial and utilized in every diagnosis, taking into consideration factors like Qi, yin, and yang and the five element theory.

According to the face-reading time line the practice of face reading was developed at the time of 220 B.C. and was documented in the earliest Bamboo Chronicles In (481-221 BC) Gui-Gu Tze, a well-known face-reading philosopher, wrote a book titled"Xiang Biam Wei Mang" "Xiang Biam Wei Maang". The book discusses the art of reading faces by analyzing the shape and color that the facial features. The face is composed of one or more five elements, each with an yin and Yang side. The face is composed of an average of 108 points that indicate the health of the person. According to Gui Gu Tze "To understand the skill of reading faces one needs to master the Bagua and be aware of what each symbol represents.

In the Confucius period, Chinese face reading spread throughout China, Japan, India and Korea. Face reading was a phenomenon in Europe but it was called Physiognomy. In 1272, the author Michael Scott wrote a book "The Hominis Physiognomia" and in the early 1700's an Swiss pastor known by the name of Johann Lavater wrote an in thorough article on the art of reading faces. In 1750, a man named Nanboku Mizuno, a native of Japan became famous for his technique of physiognomy. In the last few years, George Oshawa was inspired by Dr. Sagen Ishizuka in the 1900s and wrote a book on the use of face reading to assess the diet of a person based on their appearance. In the 1970s, one of George Oshawa's became famous throughout the world as the most accurate facial reader in the day. Charles Yarborough wrote an article on the basic principles of face reading, using the ancient theories to analyze the art. This time-line clearly shows the significance and effectiveness of the technique and continues to be used as an effective diagnostic tool to this day.

Quoted by"The Yellow Emperor:

Chinese facial reading is Diagnostic Tool

Treatise 17

In the "Treatise on the importance of the Pulse as well as the subliminal Skill of its Examining" The Yellow Emperor was interested in knowing what procedure an examiner follows when watching patients when conducting an exam. He was provided with the below: "The medical treatment should be performed at dawn, in the morning when Yin (feminine energy) has not yet begun to rise and when Yang (male energy) is not yet awake, when there is nothing that has been eaten, there is not enough energy in the 12 major vessels (Jing Mo) and when the lovessels (Luo Mo) are awaken in a state where force and energy are not disturbed, that is when the pulse is taken. Five colors as well as the colors of the eyes must be observed in order to see"Shen "Shen" of the person. This includes observing excessive or inadequate, and regardless of whether six bowels appear strong or weak. The body's appearance should be declining or improving. After all five tests are completed, the results must be compared". This demonstrates the importance of observation during an examination, which is being followed to this day. It also indicates the ideal time to look at and determine the condition of a patient since you have to take into consideration the yin and the yang that are present in the current day. Examining the face and the colour of the skin can indicate the time when illness is present and what organs are affected.

Chapter 6: What Do Chinese Face Reading Determine Illness within the body?

The Context of "Ming Chiang" "...

The classification of the Constitution can be observed through the face, based on theory of yin and Yang that are supported by the five elements theory. Every organ can be identified by the geometric form of the face. It determines the shape and dimensions of organs. If you are giving advice on health to patients or educating them about the illness, it can be useful if it is given using the tongue or through pulse diagnosis. These fundamental properties of generalization could be powerful when applied to every concept like personal characters as well as physiology, toxicology, and the pulse diagnosis.

If we examine the body and face we can observe the Qi that is the vital force that drives every living thing. Mien Shiang believes that perfect facial proportions and balance indicates the person will experience luck, health, wealth and happiness. Yang and yin represent the mountains and the valley of the face. Symmetry and proportion are crucial because they represent a simple life route.

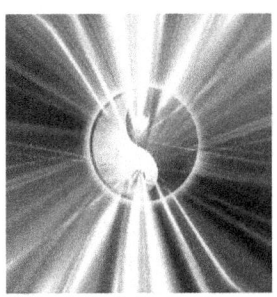

The yin portion of the face is the valley that has soft characteristics like the soft, smooth and fluid elements in the face. The yang component is the mountains that make up the face like the sharp and hard components in the facial structure. The yang components of the face include the chin, forehead jaw bones, cheek bones, which comprise the tissues that are hard on the face. The face's yin areas include the ears, nose and cheeks. They include the chin, chin, mouth, eyes and the tip of the nose, which are fluid facial features. When yin and Yang change the appearance of the face is affected due to emotions, age or physical trauma. One strives to achieve the harmony of two, however the balance between yin and Yang is constantly changing , and balance is rarely attained.

Chinese Emperors were adept at their art Chinese faces reading. It was the Chinese emperor Qin Shi Huang which was the first ruler of China in 221 B.C. defeated the art of Mien-Shiang and the entire written literature on his art Chinese face reading, as and his official portrait. He then created a fake image of himself that incorporated all the traits of Mien Shiang, which demonstrates his positive qualities. He painted the perfect picture of love and a good ruler. The world watched him when he painted the perfect picture for them to follow.

In the modern world of research, face reading is still widely used. When we meet someone we are innately influenced about the person. In our minds, we are able to read the person's body the way they talk, their personality and even their face. Barak Obama, the President of America United States has a wood element face. There have been many other presidents before him. Chinese faces have shown that people tend to follow a face made of wood. People who aren't experts may not grasp the significance of face reading, but it's more effective than most people believe.

When we learn to interpret facial expressions to determine health issues, we can help our patients with greater efficiency and provide them with advice about changing their habits. The shape, color, and lines could indicate diseases that are related to specific organs. The ancient art of facial expression, if studied and understood, can help our health as it did hundreds of years ago. The face represents our present, past and the future. If certain ailments are evident by the appearance of the face treatment may be offered to alter the future health of the patient. Classical texts have shown the importance of the basic understanding of philosophy and how it impacts us today.

To master how to master Chinese face reading, it's essential to study with an expert, but one must be aware that some face reading instructors charge high charges for readings that contain incorrect details. It is crucial to do some research about facial readers and discover the details that are available online or in publications. I think people in the west will greatly benefit from the use of this instrument to aid in health tests. Your face is your way of communicating with the outside world, and researchers believe that emotions influence us. Unfortunately, the western world is still unaware of this ancient practice. Being an TCM practitioner will open you up to an entire world of information, and guides you in becoming the best within the TCM world.

What are The Principles of Chinese Face Reading?

Chinese face reading is a combination of the both the yin and the yang as well as the five element theory. It also incorporates the past, present and the future and also your internal organs. The balance and proportions are important.

The face is comprised of three quarters, eight trigrams, and 108 zones. The 108 areasrepresent the lines that are created throughout our lives. The wrinkles moles, color spots, and wrinkles are usually located along these lines, or in close proximity to them, and each has the meaning behind them.

The shape and the color of the face to determine whether there is a problem within the body, as the appearance of the face may be related to certain ailments.

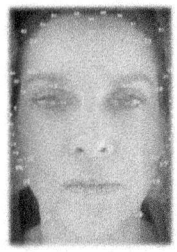

The premise behind Chinese face reading is that it reveals the emotional, spiritual, and mental aspects of an individual. The face can reveal a lot of information about an individual without asking any questions. Based on this information, we can assess the state of health of the organs and the way they affect them when it is evident in the facial color.

What are the 5 different types of faces?

The facial shape

The five face kinds are closely related to the five element theory that includes earth, fire water, metal and wood. The face's shape is closely related to the elements, which give us information about the health of a patient. The face's shape will reveal the personality of a person's nature, their weaknesses as well as the diseases that can impact the face. In the past, each face was made up of one element, however in the course of time, this has changed and the majority of faces are elements that are mixed. This is evidently a reflection of life because the conflict of elements creates conflict and the changes that occur that we experience in our lives.

The eyes are considered to be eyes that are the "door to the heart". The Chinese believes that when the eyes shine and sparkle, people have a strong heart-spirit, and a weak one when eyes seem dull. This diagram clearly outlines the components that are related to the organs and the associated organs that are affected.

Element Organ hollow organs

Wood Liver Gallbladder

Fire Heart Small Intestine

Metal Lung Large Intestine

Water Kidney Bladder

Earth Spleen Stomach

The Wood Face

The face of the wood could be described as A long nose and face with a wide forehead, with slim cheeks. The eyes look nice and hair tends to be thick. The eyebrows would be long and big. The real signification of wood is its high and broad forehead. This wood feature indicates expansion, future growth as well as the plan and vision of a plan. Growth and maturity are important character traits. They tend to be leaders, organizers and individuals with strong thoughts.

The path they take in life is thrown away by growth and achievement This is the way of their lives that allows them to discover the more they know about themselves. The challenges of this face show the lack of flexibility and their overly smug views. The wood face is afflicted by anger person the most since they tend to be strong-headed and are unable to take failure as a sign of not controlling their emotions. People can be frustrated by intense anger, also known as the yang element or fall into depression called the yin aspect. The theory is that when a tree is not able to develop or grow new twigs, it becomes angry, confused and angry.

If the energy flow is blocked, the gallbladder and liver that are that are affected by this element become ill within the body. Common symptoms aredigestive issues headaches, ulcers, headaches premenstrual stress, and gallstones.

The SHAPE OF A Wood FACE

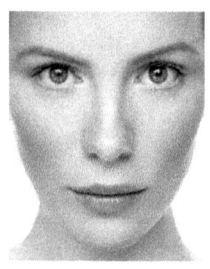

The Fire Face

The fire face is described as having a long face that has clear, thin check bones, that appear to be appearing to be sticking out, with a strong straight chin, and a forehead. The typical fire face has curly, red or wet hair, with freckles appearing on their face. They may be swift in their movements and speaking. They are known as friendly people who have an inexhaustible spark of enthusiasm and inspiration that can affect people around them in a positive manner. People with these traits typically are extremely energetic and enthusiastic. They have goals to achieve and are involved in reaching them.

The energy that is ablaze can push the person to take risky actions that they typically wouldn't but the adrenaline and excitement pushes them to take risks. People with this type of energy can be identified in asking them few life questions. The downside of this flame is that the individual may become depressed due to the lack of motivation or enthusiasm. The spark is usually gone and it is visible in their personality. They have a difficult time to keep the joy in check and the warmth inside.

If the fire is suffocated or overactive, the heart is extremely affected. The heart is controlled by the fire and the small intestine. They are often required to take nutrients for blood. They are afflicted by anxiety, heart conditions, and insomnia as well as skin eruptions. The heart also controls the mind which can cause restless nights and stress.

The design and shape of the Fire Face

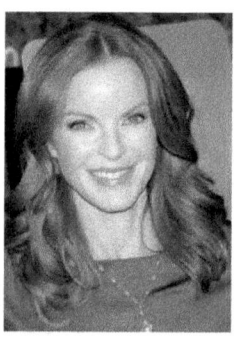

The Earth Face

The face of the earth is defined by a short, square face with the jawline being distinct. Earth face people typically have deep voices, and are usually of a large build and have massive bones. They have a pale complexion and typically possess larger features on their face, for example, the mouth or lips. Earth faces have the ability to feel relaxed and in touch with within. They also have the capacity to live a happy life on a solid base.

Their traits show that they are trustworthy and dependable. They are also practical. They are prudent with their spending and consider their choices before making decisions. They are rational and are not as emotional as people who drink water. They're very traditional. The problems they confront are usually related to food related issues. The stomach and spleen control this aspect, which could be the reason they suffer from food-related issues or diseases that cause them to be unable to make flow and suffer from a lack of Qi or energy. Earth types are aware of the importance of their diet and the way of life.

They recognize the importance of good health by including digestive enzymes and supplements in their diet. They should avoid dairy and sugar as they can cause dampness in the body, which in turn creates mucus within the connective tissue. Patients often complain of swelling, weight gain in the legs and the body. They may be tired and sluggish often. If a patient doesn't have a jaw line but an earth-like face, we are able to detect that the patient has an issue with their jaw because the jaw line is closely connected to stomach meridian.

The earth's shape face

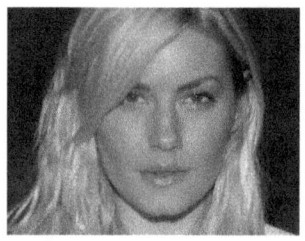

The metal face

The face of the metal is defined by a square form with prominent cheekbones and light white skin. They're usually very attractive looking and have bright, glowing eyes. They are straight with light eyebrows and a cut speech. In the corporate world, they're often excellent counselors, lawyers, or advisors. They are also effective as healers, teachers or tutors.

Personality-wise, they are powerful, wild and troublesome. They are a bit routine-oriented and possess strong tendencies. They have a sense of humor and generally have a positive outlook on life. Also, they have a committed attitude to life. They're not afraid of doing their best. A metal's negative traits face are negative thoughts that affect their mental health in a negative way. They are very responsive to alternative treatments. In order to be content, they must be imaginative. It is important to imagine them as metal. When metal starts to rust it is a sign that there is no joy and when the metal shines with brightness , it indicates that they are satisfied. It is essential for people to be able to express their feelings.

Depression is often a cause of respiratory system problems or lower gastrointestinal diseases. The face of metal is governed by the lungs and the large the intestine. It is essential to include breathing exercises into their lives as illness is likely to affect these regions first. It is essential to establish an ideal lifestyle since food items that are unhealthy will be taken in with health issues.

The design on the surface of the steel

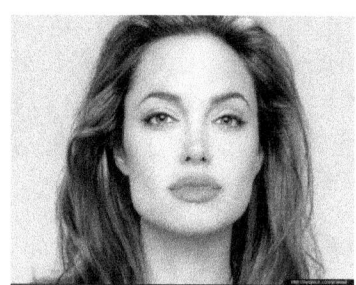

The water face

A water face is identified by a round-face, often seen as being overweight. They usually have big eyes, however they have softness and care for darker hair and skin. They are usually described as emotional because they are quiet, sensitive and delicate. They have a difficult time managing their emotions and you can clearly see when they are unhappy or upset. Because of their sensitive nature, they are extremely adept in storytelling and are excellent communicaters.

Their sensitivity makes them adept listeners, counselors, and caregivers. Water faces are often intuitive, and they are described as magnets since they pull what they require immediately. They are aware of the things they want and move to get it. To understand them, it is important to imagine the water. Water that is clear flows freely, making the water flexible. If the water is stagnant , then unrepressed emotions can cause dark circles and blue tinges under the eyes , which is related to kidneys.

Water face linked to the kidneys as well as the bladder, which results in excessive soft tissues and deeply rooted emotions that affect the tissues very profoundly. Water can become irritable or stressed, as well as overworked because of kidney yin deficiency. This can cause an internal heat, which triggers the swelling of inflammation in the body.

The design that the Water Face

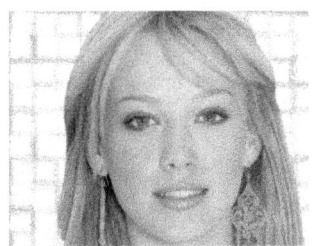

What is the color of the Face signifies?

This article will help you in making the most accurate diagnosis by simply observing the facial color.

Color Significance

The skin is yellow in color. Insufferable digestion

A dull and shiny face. Weak immunity or poor lung function

Face swelling Damp inside the body

Dark blue tinges appear under the eyes. The eyes are affected by adrenal and kidney imbalance, as well as over work

Puffy forehead swollen with lines. Excessive intake of oily rich and oily foods

Redness Poor circulation or heart disease and high blood pressure inflammation

Green, yellow and blue minerals deficiency due to lower the function of the liver

Your health is determined by your appearance

Every feature on the face corresponds to an organ in accordance with Traditional Chinese Medicine. This can be an effective tool to use during an appointment. Discoloration and lines does not only signify illness, it can also be a sign of an organ. Following the consultation, the most frequent symptom distinction will be Qi which is blood deficiency an imbalance of yin and Yang, as well as blood stasis.

If your ears are affected it means that the kidneys aren't functioning properly, however it is also possible to have excess. This is why it's crucial to have a complete consult to review all details before formulating the treatment program. The table below shows the facial area that is linked to various organs in the body.

Chapter 7: Face Reading

You don't know your face in the same way you know! The first step to identifying emotions on other people is to be aware of what's happening on your appearance is.

We all share the same muscles on our face, males, females and children, no matter if they are they are in Outer Mongolia or inner Birmingham. It has been proven the existence of seven emotions states that are visible on the face of the human being and are common to everyone.

They are instinctual and not learned. Certain facial muscles and , consequently, emotional faces are simple to pull out of the blue and consequently make up. Certain facial muscles that are involved with particular expressions are difficult or impossible to be activated voluntarily by the majority of people, and are therefore especially reliable when interpreting other people's facial expressions.

Yes, you have a good idea of the way people communicate with you through subconsciously reading the facial muscles of their faces, and the forehead in particular and that's what top actors and actresses, as well as numerous politicians have either discovered or already knew to be the case.

The biggest problem with your knowledge is the face of your own.

Be aware of your types

What is an Macro? :

The most common phrases run between 1/2-second between 4 and 1/2-seconds. We frequently repeat them and they work with what we're saying as well as the tone and pitch of our voice.

What is a micro? :

These are a fleeting appearance, visible on our faces between 1/15 to 1/25 of one second. They are the result of suppressing or repressing emotions that we may want to cover up or are unaware of in the absence of conscious awareness.

What is a False Statement? :

This is a deliberate effort to mimic an emotion and show the emotion through the eyes.

What's a Masked/Squelched expression? :

This is a false statement designed to disguise macro-expressions in order to disguise it. Then, why and when are Micro Expressions occur?

They happen when we block the emotions we feel by preventing them from fully being expressed. The reason for this is twofold such as Repression (when we aren't conscious of or do not recognize the beginning of an emotional state) or Suppression (when we are conscious of the onset of an emotion, but try to hide that emotion from being noticed by others.

Are they Suppressing, Expressing or Repressing?

Importantly, both instances are similar in the sense that one is unable to discern whether the phrase itself is the result that is the result of suppression (deliberate concealment) or the other way around: repression (unconscious concealment) This is the root of many debates and confusion.

Then it's the responsibility of your cross-referencing skills to determine whether someone is conscious or subconsciously hiding their feelings.

You Don't Know What's On Your Face Is Doing

The face of ours is constantly communicating. It has been proven scientifically that certain expressions evoke certain emotions and are ingrained in our bodies. When you finish this book, you'll find the image of a tiny girl expressing a look of delight. We don't really understand what we are saying to other people most times. We look at our reflection to know why someone would tell us something like, "stop staring at me this way or "please get that look off your face!', or 'you might remain like that or something like that, the expression will have been discarded. The good news is that the majority of people don't realize what their faces are doing all the time, and it's all around for anyone who is interested to easily read!

It is the same with every face, regardless the age. It is possible that you can't recognize these expressions in this short period of time. To begin you'll have to take a look at photos and slower motion, or freeze frames. But, you are able to quickly train your mind to detect them, and in no time you'll be aware of the expressions. You've always noticed these, even though you've never been aware of it. This book will help bring awareness of them.

Do You Want to Be Reputable?

There are many variations that can be seen in the faces of humans. even the faces of identical twins can change with time, as we weave the range of emotions and state into the facial canvas. The way we communicate and the gestures we use differ greatly between cultures and when it comes to our polite social interactions, we frequently don't mean the words we use or what we are saying for a variety of appropriate social reasons.

The face, however, is a universal set of signs that show changes in emotions from moment to moment and is completely reliable. It is astonishment the fact that as I said and I will say that we don't actually know what is happening to our faces are up to.

Know Your Face!

I'll also predict that after you've achieved the art of being able to let yourself feel genuine anger and then actually capturing your face with that expression by lifting the mirror or filming yourself and replaying it frame-by-frame it is likely that you will display more often! It is possible to practice your "surprised" face in order to be a good looking host at the unexpected party you be aware of!

I am currently enthralled at the reasons why women spend a significant quantity of their time the layers upon layers of makeup that are only used to enhance the unattractive look of their face. It truly makes you realize that the best way to appear appealing is to have an expression of happiness.

I've had many gorgeous women in my courses of training who are astonished by the sight of photos of the group , which shows their faces in a state of discontent as they wrestle with an idea. Are you aware of what the expression of your face when you're angry, or what anger that I see? Perhaps it's disgust. It is commonly misinterpreted as anger.

In addition, I've found it is true because we're so poor at distinguishing fake smiles from genuine one, when you attempt to brighten up your face and your day by smiling at others (smiling rather than just smiles without a reason this is!) The majority of people will be able to smile back, and your fake smile transforms into a real one.

The ability to discern microexpressions will allow you to identify the emotions of other people (particularly in cases where they don't recognize they are expressing them) and simultaneously you'll be more conscious of your own emotions and be able to cut off negative emotions in the bud. You can do things to make your mood better If you wish to! You might be a fan of letting yourself indulge in the occasional bout of misery and would like a little empathy and maybe you'd be denial of your humanity at least every now and then at the very minimum!

Do You Want to be an Mind Reader?

Every interaction you have are enhanced by these abilities. I've often been described as a mind reader or infused with psychic powers because I can detect emotional states and then address them. Since I am a certified trainer, I have believed this to be a must.

I think I acquired my abilities through a long period of reactions to thousand of people and hundreds of facial expressions. perhaps my talents were born out of the desire to control emotional outbursts before they got too overwhelming to bear! Most people are somewhat sensitive in the event that their daily jobs were set to be drastically altered by an introduction to a computerized system they were unsure of how to utilize.

Technology and tantrums could be gone forever but I am sure there are other things that cause anxiety now.

The state of our emotions is an important factor in all interactions. The macro expressions don't accurately reflect how a person is experiencing. This is because you are aware of how easy it is to hide how you're experiencing!

Through these techniques to improve your skills, you'll be more skilled in recognizing when emotions are just beginning or when it is concealed and when a person isn't aware of the emotions they're experiencing, which is interesting to think about. To be aware of the state of mind of another person before they can recognize it in their own mind and to effectively and with tact upon that knowledge is a great skill indeed. You'll know that you've been lied to, even if you do not be aware of the reason, and the "why" is vital. This is highly confidential information. Make use of it with care.

Do You Want to Identify Hidden Emotions?

Are you confident enough to go through with this? Because, keep in mind that I won't be able to 'put back' you once you've figured it out! If you recognize an expression and are able to determine the meaning, it's your choice how you apply the information, whether you cross-reference by asking questions or letting the expression go. We call it an unconscious "leakage" whenever someone tries to conceal or control emotions as the unconscious, which is the one responsible for all your bodily functions , such as breathing and beating your heart and will usually activate a muscle related to the emotion that is evident on that person's appearance.

It may be limited to a specific area on the face (a subdued expression) or it could be a flashy expression that is flashed across the face (a micro-expression).

Do You Want Better Relationships?

When you learn to recognize the things your face is like and be able to recognize and address the emotional states of other people and your relationships will greatly improve. It's possible to have to go through testing first, but.

Your friends are adept at being able beguile you, distract you, and disarm you when you let things go by your way. They do the same to you as well. We all require our own space and a unique method of keeping certain items private. Research has also revealed that people who were able to recognize facial expressions in micro scales were observed to be more appreciated by their colleagues in their environments. This understanding and awareness will help you better comprehend and effectively the other people around you, and to be able to comprehend what your facial expressions are giving information about your internal moods.

Stop thinking you know what others are thinking.

Studies have shown that we tend to miss facial expressions that contradict the words spoken. It appears that we are more responsive to what is being said rather than the expressions that the face can offer. Everybody has a face and everybody utilizes it in specific ways when they are experiencing the seven distinct emotions. Therefore, you aren't able to comprehend the other person, and more specifically than that, you totally miss the mark when you believe you understand them. And that's the issue to the vast majority all of the interactions we have!

In the future we may find that research might provide more established states to determine however seven is sufficient for this moment.

This means you can see the faces of people who come from different cultures, who don't speak your language . In the actuality how many times have you had to interact with a foreigner in another country and was able to convey your sadness or joy, anger, sadness, etc. and have been accepted and assisted?

Everyone has the same emotions and show the same emotions. It is important to realize that it's not only what you hear that's significant, it's what you see and they must connect for people to be consistent in their communications. Oddly enough, we are at a loss and tolerant when someone voiced an disagreement with our preconceived notions for example"I told you, I'm fine! We know that they're not do we?

Control your mood and be happier

We have learned this in our classes over time and it is now a to be a fact that changing the facial expression to an expression that is well-known can trigger the physiological response of the emotion. You must be prepared for this since we have discovered that by being in the expression of anger or sadness for any amount in time, thought patterns that are related to the state of mind are able to enter your mind and in the nick of time, you may really be in a sad!

Be sure to close with a big, old smile or with someone you are able to be with and laugh with. One of the most exciting benefits of being able to read faces of other people is that you will begin to recognize your own face moving in specific directions.

This is all without the need to have a mirror in the first place It's like we start to recognize the moment when expressions are developing and we begin to recognize our triggers and create a positive response instead of being in a strong condition that is difficult to get from.

Moody Momentum

It is possible to be overwhelmed and be too consumed to be able to get out. This usually happens when we know we're in a state of anger or frustration and someone else reflects the same sentiment back at us (anger can spread quickly, and misery definitely loves company). It's like we've entered the worst mood and we would like the people in our surroundings to be in the same mood and we're not happy until they're. Take a moment to think about this second.

Consider a time in your life when you were actually, irritated by something, but the person you were with did not comprehend the annoyance, and instead advises you to let this go'. Or says they are unable to comprehend the reason you're so angry. The majority of human beings desire to be understood more than anything other things even at the expense of their mental health So the downward spiral starts.

The fact that we are instructed to smile and forget it can help. The cheeriness of other people only increases our despair or anger. That's where the ferocity of your energetic state holds held you so strongly that the only option is to simply take it on. Once you've recollected and recognize this that the person telling lies is on on a wave of energy and all you need to do is to make an accusation that you don't believe you and then all hell will be released. Also, you're missing important details that you might need.

If you are able to catch yourself in the initial surge of anger or sadness and see it appear on your face , you can become more curious and be aware of it. Then opt to be focused on something other than that! By letting go of the distractions of your surroundings, the softness of a cushion or the smell of a weed growing on the asphalt or the sound of music that you hear in a bustling supermarket or a smile of gratitude from an old man walking across the road in the rain while you take in the comfort of your car as you stand at the pedestrian crossing and you are able to pull yourself away from the mood to stop momentum from from building. The real magic happens when you feel the first flash of emotion on the face of a loved one and disperse any momentum and end a fight that's developing.

Many times, I people come from work with a bad mood and the energy builds and continues to grow through the night until it is not getting released at the boss or anyone else who caused the resentment, that negative mood manifests itself in the comfort and warmth at home, with the people we love most.

Make a promise to yourself that you'll be looking at every day, especially the mirror in the rear view, or the bathroom mirror, and be aware of the way your face communicates in all its moody state and then begin to form an connection of the way your face appears with what you feel. The people you love will be grateful to for your efforts.

Do You Want Friends?

Being aware of what your appearance is doing, and knowing how to speak up about those behaviors to others, or be able to recognize them and alter the subject rapidly(!) can greatly assist in developing social abilities.

Chapter 8: Analysis of Deception And You

Recent research on deceit revealed the existence of seven micro-expressions that are fleeting and 'subtle expressions' (where only a specific portion of the face showing the expression) which result from suppressing intense feelings.

Now You Know It, But You Don't

So, as you already know, a microexpression is recorded on the face within a microsecond. They are distinct when compared to facial expressions because we don't really enjoy the way we display them (either conscious or not) and they fade quickly.

You've often picked the signs without having a conscious awareness of them. And when you become conscious of something that is not right, the phrase is gone, and you begin to question your own intuition. You did notice them but until you're aware of what they mean or you are fortunate enough to witness slowed-down footage of the expression to prove your suspicions, you're uncertain.

The only thing you can be certain about is your face which you are able to slow down however you'd like when you look when you look in the mirror! It is safe to let the rest of it to your subconscious mind to see the faces of others since you can't perform this task consciously because the expressions are too quick.

Micro expressions are a part of the totality of the face, and utilize the same muscles of the face of every one of us. The subtle expressions are part of the muscles and are usually indicators of a full emotional state. Learn to read people by understanding your own facial expressions.

What are the reasons and why do they When and Why Do They

The subtle and micro-expressions of the face are scientifically proven to be the hidden emotions that can be seen on the face during high-risk situations where there is something significant to lose or gain from the event of a crisis.

They are triggered when a person is consciously or unconsciously hiding the intensity of a feeling. The scientifically-proven to be seven emotions that have universal messages across the faces of all humans that include: joy; sadness, anger, fear as well as disgust, surprise and disdain. Images of every expression and, consequently the state of each emotion at the end of this book.

When these expressions flash on the face in the span of one second, you literally blink, and then you are missing these expressions. You don't even notice them conscious of it, even though your subconscious has been aware of them for years and has been taught from an early age on how to react to these expressions.

Now, Get Your Face Ready

Get your mirror and switch on your webcam to ensure you'll be capable of seeing your face clearly.

Get ready for your appearance. This may sound somewhat silly. In reality, it should read maybe "Don't get your face ready'. Take a moment to think of times when you've observed your face without the effort you put into to it prior to your seeing! That's right, when someone has snapped an image of you doesn't suit you or when you spot your reflection in a window of a shop such as. Also, in the present, when the camera on your phone is turned upside down as you view your face in a strangely-angled angle looking at the camera.

I was a bit confused when I stepped into that tiny metal box, instead of the stunning scene that you believed you were taking pictures of!

A fun experiment that will surprise you.

Prior to looking at your image, take a moment to relax your face. Relax all muscles of your cheeks, forehead jaw, and chin. It's quite a talent to let everything go, however, try it.

Then, literally, without moving any muscle or even your face take a look at your face with a keen eye.

If you are able to take your face in the way it appears to be at peace It is now time to note the features of your face and without judgement.

Take a deep breath and imagine some sad thing. How do you imagine it could occur to your forehead? What do you think could be happening on your eyebrows? Really think of something painful to you personally. And then, only then, close your eyes and look at your reflection.

It is common that we're so shocked or even apathetic to our own expression that we alter the expression 'automatically'. In the event that this occurs, try the same experiment.

Take a look at my forehead and see the picture of sorrow at the end of this book. However, you should be aware that these expressions may be exaggerated to give an accurate picture of the movement of the forehead. In other words my forehead isn't as wrinkled (okay that's true however, aren't we all lucky to have such an obvious instance? Praise the events that led to wrinkles like these to assist you today!).

In sad times, the muscles of the forehead create a tendency for the eyebrows to raise towards the corners of the forehead as they experience a central lift of the forehead. It is a central lifting and is distinct from other expressions that you'll learn that require the whole forehead. The eyelids are also pulled as well, but one important aspect to note is that it is all due to the forehead muscles responding to your emotions.

Are They Truly Truthful or Not?

The people who seek to get empathy from us, either intentionally or not, tend to shift their face into this posture but you'll be able to discern the genuine sadness of an expression that is forced.

One of the best ways to learn these phrases is to do it in the comfort at home through watching replays of interview clips by expert presenters, and then looking out for the tricky question. If you can use a slow motion or freeze-frame option on the replay it's helpful. Take a look at the same interview without sound and see if you are able to identify awkward moments.

You're seeking an instantaneous flash of expressionand not prolonged frozen expression. If the expression is sustained for longer than it should it's probably not real.

Your Amazing Secret Tip No.1 :

What time did the expression appear? Was the expression noticed prior to speaking or at the start of their conversation? Micro-expressions are fleeting. They flash across your face and are often squelched the flashes. This is the term used for hiding the true expression by quickly changing it into an acceptable expression. Therefore, a genuine expression of sadness will usually be visible present on the face for only just a few seconds before disappearing.

This is typically the case that someone will say something to switch the topic or, in some cases, you alter the subject on your own, after realizing that the person you're speaking to feels uncomfortable for example"How would you like an iced tea or what? This is also when someone asks whether you're okay and you say you are. Then they move closer before asking slow, "Are you sure, are you certain you're okay?"

This is when we make great efforts to convince others that we really are "FINE," (in my experience, when someone employs the term fine, it's typically the case when there is no way to be) or when one falls into an emotional state, abandoning the pretense and accepting that one is 'found out'. The choice is usually based on your relationship with the person you are communicating with, as well as levels of trust with the person you are communicating with and, most importantly your mood!

Your Ultimate Secret Tips No.2 :

The face remains fixed when the expression is too long. We know instinctively that these expressions will disappear (unless you are witnessing someone breaking into massive rage or despair, and even then the expression shifts, maybe by hiding their face and squirting various secretions using an emery board) which is why it's unusual to see the forehead frozen in this way. There is no time limit for you to decide the length of time this should take but you'll be able to tell.

Your Amazing Secret Tip No.3 :

Other facial features starts to be a part of the picture! Sometimes, the lips' corners droop down by themselves.

We have learned to spot the expressions on our faces in the way they appear, often the mouth isn't joined and it can be the mouth, and more so than the forehead! This would be an innocuous expression rather than an expression that is micro. That's why they are not rigid and quick rules. These are suggestions that you can cross-reference by asking questions or keeping a record of in your own head and then revisiting in the future.

What did your face do? What did you do to your muscles in your forehead, brows and eyes?

Chapter 9: Learn More Details About Your Amazing Forehead

Be aware of your forehead's muscles

If you've ever witnessed your own skull on the x-rays or seen your physical self' on an MRI scan, or similar it's a wake-up call to see what's going on beneath the skin that we think for so much. We are obsessed with cleansing, moisturising and tanning. There are muscles within your face, and we can learn some facts about the muscles. Muscles can be cardiac, non-striated or striated

The muscles that are strenuous are connected to bones, and give us the freedom to exercise voluntarily moving i.e. we have control over it. When we frown or smile in general, we can control the movement with our muscles.

Non-striated muscles (also called smooth muscles) tend to be involuntary, and they work in a way that is automatic.

There are many muscles that make up the facial muscles. They enable people to move their facial muscles to create expressions and communicate. The facial muscles play an crucial in speech.

Your 43 facial muscles and 3,000 expressions!

There are believed as 43 facial muscles that can produce 3,000 facial expressions that are meaningful WOW. We'll only be looking at a handful of reliable certain ones.

here!

Make-up artists working in the film industry employ makeup to express emotion or enhance the character's appearance e.g. applying lines or shading to the brows can create emotion, sadness or anger.

If a woman exaggerates her appearance to make herself make her appear attractive, it's those particular features that are exaggerated and appear a bit sexy in the event that her face gets drawn into a slouching stance.

Try this: put enormous amounts of makeup on your lips and eyes and then be extremely angry about something, then take a look at yourself at yourself in the mirror! Don't make me feel guilty that I'm male. This is just an experiment! Consider the most disgusting thing you can possibly put in your mind. Then, multiply that sentiment by 100. then look at yourself. Ugh. Imagine the most frightening thing you could possibly come across think of, or what is the most frightening to you in your life. Then take the look!

Expressions of the Forehead

Every expression has forehead counterparts, but some are more noticeable within that region. There are shades in the seven major expressions and there are a variety of expressions, including shock, worry and apprehension and sadness all appearing on the forehead. If you inquire as to what the person has been doing and a sly expression flashes across the forehead, it's best to study the situation and discover the reason for this extreme reaction. It is possible that the person simply be scared of not believing them , or perhaps annoyed that you would even inquire But what you're seeking is the emotion , and to identify the root of the issue.

The muscles of the forehead create facial expressions. There are four fundamental movements of the forehead that may occur when combined to create various expressions.

The muscles that raise the eyebrows are called the occipitofrontalis muscles, whether in tandem or independently, creating expressions of shock and awe. The corrugator supercilii muscles be used to pull the eyebrows backwards and downwards, creating an expression of frowning on the face. The procerus muscles are able to draw down the middle portion of the eyebrows to create the appearance of a frown.

I've included photos of our foreheads resting in the pictures relevant to the end of the book to make it easier for you to compare.

The Angry, The Fearful and the Surprised

Pay attention to the inner corner of your eyebrow and the arch that is on each side in the expression you are reading, whether it's in the real world or from photographs in this book.

Do it yourself, pull your eyebrows down dramatically in the inner corners. What sensation does this create in you? If your lips are tight to the point of narrowing, and if your cheeks are pushed up then you've definitely made it! This is certainly an expression of anger.

In the photos of shock take note of the upward lift over the whole brow, and the overall smooth upward arches.

Now, what you need to look out for is the difference. It is recognizing these differences which will provide clues to the emotion that is being expressed on the face or in the photo. Are the eyebrows pulled up or down? Then, observe if the lines on the forehead are arched and smooth, or slightly sharp, bringing the eyebrows in an uneven pattern, as could be a sign of the cause of fear.

Active Expression, Neutral

If you then look at the various foreheads you're around What do you think and can you determine what is which? Look for jaggedness or smoothness and, remember, the expressions appear the same across all faces regardless of race, gender or age. If someone is lying to you, they could be afraid of having their lie accepted or frightened that they're not telling the truth, and that you might not believe them.

First, before thinking that a face that is lined is angry, or something else ensure that you calibrate your camera: are aware of the face you're reading in its neutral condition before you try to interpret an emotion. Try it out on your own face , using a mirror or a webcam. It is essential to remain neutral initially before you begin to feel emotions running through your body and observe your face's expression. Snapping a photo is the best option since you'll be able to analyze it later on, before the effect fades! You have the right to make the selfie taken.

It is also evident that if you hold your face with the position for a long time it is when you begin experiencing the feeling, and your thoughts will be entangled with memories of the emotion you experienced. So, you should ensure you finish your sentence with a an optimistic smile to clear the slate.

Battle of Darwin vs Mead Battle of Darwin Versus Mead

Darwin declared that all mammals display emotions on their faces. This was stated by him in "The Expression of emotions in Man as well as Animals" in 1872.

Then, there was Margaret Mead in the 1960s. She believed that the expressions we use are culturally influenced and thus learned behavior, determined by the environment and our reactions to them.

Real Smiles vs False Smiles and Real Sadness

In bringing us back to the practicality of current applications of this work at a fundamental level it's interesting for all of us to be able to determine and not guess whether an emotion is real or fake. The easiest thing to fake is the smile. The lower portion of the face in an image and then take a look at their eyes. Are the eyes smiling often in photographs of celebrities, it's just the mouth that is making the correct shape, and is actually a fake beautiful, but fake smile. It is impossible to stop a genuine smile, since studies have revealed the genuine smile that appears on faces of suspects when a police officer pretends to believe that lies are being told.

One of the most skeptics among all facial expressions, the smile. You've always been aware that the smile is not an authentic smile. Your subconscious will have noticed the fact that your eyes aren't aligned with the efforts of the other facial features!

Automated expressions, or expressions that engage the facial muscles without conscious thought, rather than through conscious, deliberate actions can be characterized as sad. A sad-looking face shows the inner corner of your eyebrow rises, but not the entire eyebrow. Studies have revealed that just 15% of people is able to do this freely and thus sadness is one of the most reliable emotional facial expressions that can be read.

At this point, that some muscles are difficult to activate and sometimes impossible for most people to be activated without conscious thought. This makes certain movements more reliable than other ones.

Chapter 10: Fear is It's Hard To Create

The most effective facial muscles are located on the forehead, but when you are angry, there is an additional signal that is reliable of a closing of the lips. When you're scared, your forehead and brows are slightly uplifted and jagged, and it is very difficult to fake. You can tell when you're near to the fact that you don't want anyone to know when you notice fears.

In my personal experience I've seen numerous flashes of anger and of fear on faces (soon suppressed, especially for women in which anger isn't socially acceptable) that are reflected by a jutting jaw or a pushed upwards the chin that can cause the lips to sag.

It is further aggravated by women who wear very bold lipstick and shining as a light source to me from far away when I present issues that aren't on the shoulders of a woman who has a little. If you are able to discern the chin's shape clearly, it's evident that the thinness of the lips is caused by an upward tilt of the chin that can be a sign of anger expression. However, it is important to being aware that the thinness is not caused by the slight smile. In anger, there's movement in the middle of the chin when it is lifted up. In panic, the mouth gets tight and stretched out laterally towards the ears. This is different from the soft, relaxed lips that a genuine smile displays.

Why would someone be lying to you in order to conceal their state of mind? They might be able to sense that their emotional reaction to a particular situation is

Your personal feelings may not be the same as yours, so it's not right for them to think it.

Why would they lie to You?

Why would someone be lying to you? In any circumstance it is that they don't feel at ease expressing their true emotions. Especially in the realm of therapy as well as in the context of intimate relationships, the initial step in establishing a good relationship is to allow others to feel secure to express their feelings regardless of your opinion about their authenticity.

Therefore, sadness could be transformed into fear they fear your reaction to their mood. Faked or forced sadness may turn into an authentic smile when the person who is lying realizes that they have cheated you and hence the phrase 'duping delight', which is what you will notice when you try to believe the lie that is told to you. This is among ways to cross reference when you suspect that a child, for instance or telling you a lie. If you make it appear as if you are a believer in every word, and then you notice a slight smile, then you're busted! Wow, how a messy web we make...

Therefore, the emotion that is involved with the act of lying include:

1. Fear of being caught

2 Guilty of lying

3 Guilt over behaviour

4 Duping delight

Apart from the obvious desire to avoid being exposed as a liar and to not be caught out in a lie, the person you're talking to may not want to hear. You've always been aware that someone is not keen to discuss a topic that you've mentioned and you are not consciously directed by them to switch the topic: you start to feel uncomfortable and then you go off to turn on the kettle.

What is the Shape of Fear

Your abilities can be tested as many smiles disguise anxiety. What could appear to be an uncomfortable smile could be an lateral pulling of the corners of the lips toward the ears instead of an upward lift or a slanting of the corner. There is no way to smile with their lips a little apart and without showing teeth. Be careful, however, because when someone realizes at an unconscious degree that they're showing fear in their mouths they'll likely quickly'squelch it and smile to disguise.

They might not want to let you be aware that they are unhappy over an issue you believed was resolved because you discussed it to your perception of an agreement. In essence, if the mouth is open and there isn't a smile, even though there is some pressure in the jaw, this is the result of fear. In the case of fear, when the mouth is pulled involuntarily toward to the ears, your lips could be either closed or open. In shock the jaw and mouth relax, usually with the mouth opening.

Emotional states that are hard to define are anxiety, fear and anxiety, as well as sadness, terror and discontent. The easiest are surprise and anger.

Mouth Reading Nutshell

For you, the nutshells of and your reading of your mouth the following: a slack jaw without movement or widening its mouth is an indication of surprise; an angular chin that results from it either protruding out or extending towards the nostrils is anger. pulling from the corner of your mouth toward the ears when lips are either open or closed the natural downward drooping the mouth's corners toward the floor indicates sadness. Remember, too, that if your eyes do not join in by rolling slightly as the smile comes out then that's an indication of a false smile.

Content that can be considered offensive?

What may appear like an expression of smile, even if it isn't appropriate in the circumstances, or perhaps off-color or 'smirky' could very well be considered to be contempt. When we say contempt, it refers to an act of self-righteousness, and it is especially evident when a liar is aware of their lies are accepted.

Be aware that contempt usually can turn into a smile quickly. There aren't many people out there who are comfortable being a bit contemptuous. Ensure that you don't confuse the genuine beauty of a lopsided smile with a sneer that is contemptuous!

In a state of disdain, the entire face is raised, creating the eye slightly larger than its counterpart. And when you're aware of the thing you're seeking, you will are able to see it with incredible accuracy! This is the only face that my students are quick to recognize and make comments upon when they are first introduced to.

Usually, the expression of contempt is displayed on the face briefly, while smiling lasts for a longer time. There are instances that you see a brief smile, when someone feels they shouldn't be like the funeral smirk or fast flash of smile when one is thought to be lying. Keep in mind that these situations can be a bit out of our control, but the body is not a lie. In a truly beautiful smile the eyes are slightly smaller and identical in size, but when one eye is in disdain, it is definitely more tangled than the other!

Chapter 11: Are You Just Disgusted, Or A Psychopath?

People with psychopathic tendencies have certain ways of conducting themselves when they're lying. Although it may be difficult to identify the lie in the traditional sense but the behaviors show up are fairly easy to spot when you know the signs to look for.

While you may like to label those you don't enjoy as being psychotic, this could be an extremely serious disorder that should not be taken lightly. Some people are extremely sensitive to being dissatisfied with things and a pull-up of the mouth toward the nose is certainly and the most unattractive (particularly when you have a mouth open!) the appearance of displeasure. You shouldn't believe that your friend is a psychopath only because they're disgusted by things at times!

What Do Psychopaths Feel If They're Smiling?

1 Excitation

2 Relief from being accepted as a fact

3 Contempt

4 Pride

If you observe an amalgamation of these characteristics of emotionality in the relationship you are in, then it might be able to justify the suspicion of the relationship to be psychotic!

Beware of Automated Expressions

In fear, anxiety and fear, both eyes rise and then join. A mere 10% of people is able to do this freely according to Ekman in his study from 1992.

This information has provided the film industry as well as animators using computers with a lot of details to authenticate their characters.

This information can be used in other directions, since it can be useful to actors as well as parents, politicians medical professionals, and teachers to be aware.

What is the reason you are being deceived?

Think about what makes the best lying liar. The process of detecting deceit is a matter of two simple concepts:

What a lieder isn't aware of is because of the lack of what's happening in the face in order to give a genuine expression. Because most of us don't gaze at ourselves when we are in a state of emotional high and, in general, we're quite inept at fakeing them. This picture is one of sadness, as you can see the top of the forehead lifted, bringing up the outer edges of eyebrows.

The reason the lieder can't be faked are because most people is unable to activate certain muscles in the face intentionally or in a conscious manner.

With the most fervent will all over the world there are areas of the face that is unable to activate in conscious awareness. This is often the distinction between a great actor and a less good actor.

How to Ways of Detecting Deception

False smiles or smiling without the involvement of eyebrows or eyes is the most straightforward to begin with. Check out the web, or take a look at those photos of office gatherings in which people have to interact and are not actually enjoying it!

It is obviously not possible for a famous person to be truly content all the time to benefit us, but they frequently have trained their eyes to appear fixed in a smile. In these images that if put your hands on the lower portion of the face with your hands and look at the face, you can determine that the person was smiling simply by the eyes. If the eyes do not appear to be smiles, it's likely fake smile.

Additionally the people (of which we all are one!) frequently attempt to trick you into believing that they're okay, or even that they're happy thanks for everything with other areas of their faces to'smile'.

They might be lifting their eyebrows and pulling the lower lip forward instead of stretching their mouths to the side, or extending the mouth upwards. They could be closing their eyes or extending lips' corners however, there is something off regarding the entire situation. This is due to the fact that we're not capable of having all our facial muscles move in a precise extent on both sides of our face simultaneously.

Asymmetry

In many cases, when we fake smiles for instance, we could believe that we are looking at both sides of our face but in reality, we're not. There are people who naturally sport lopsided smiles that are charming however, in general, it's difficult to move both sides of your face in a symmetrical manner. So the more asymmetrical the more off-base generally speaking. It is crucial to assess your candidate's personality first. Take note of their face in a relaxed state and in various expressions before casting your first stone.

Evidence of Asymmetry

1 Brow is lowered in anger is stronger on left

2 Nose-wrinklings in disgust are more prominent on the right

3 Extending lips back toward ears in fear is more powerful on the right

If you feel that something isn't quite right with the face you're watching, even if it's your own face in the mirror in the bathroom You now know what to be looking for to verify your sense.

Chapter 12: The two Big Myths Of Deception Analysis

In the past, we've tended to see these two titles as signs of lying. They've been used in movies about detectives and handed down through generations. But, are they real and trustworthy? What do they mean?

"The Gaze Aversion Myth"

The gaze Aversion occurs when would like to engage in an important and serious discussion with someone, and you begin your conversations with phrases like'I'd like to talk with you' or 'We're going to have a conversation'. The other person is informed that they must be cautious or too enthusiastic in their request to be believed. they might not look at you to think about their thoughts, being nervous about the severity of the situation, or keep their face from being scrutinized by you because they don't feel secure.

An experienced lie-teller will be aware that they are expected to be able to fidget, turn their eyes, etc. and therefore will probably stare you straight in the eyes to convince you to believe them , and to determine whether you believe the lies.

There's a problem for you as a genuine person may also do this to try to convince your understanding even if that you're unlikely to trust them.

The reasons why Gaze Aversion is a problem.

1 Sadness

2 Nervousness

3 embarrassment

4 Guilt

5 Disgust

The Fidgeting Myth

Fidgetingcould mean that you want to move about in response to the fear they are experiencing whether it is due to anxiety about the severity of your appearance or simply to distract themselves from the intensity of your gaze when you look at their actions!

Do you have a view about today? I'm wondering how many schoolmasters were this wrong when they made accusations of girls and boys who are small. They could indicate that someone is not paying attention to your gaze and glancing around a bit and in a way that is awkward however it could it is also a sign that they are slightly intimidated. You don't have to feel guilt-ridden to feel at a loss and make an individual decision as to whether defending the lie causes them to feel uncomfortable or if it's you who is asking the question!

Finally, it's just bad timing.

The genuine and authentic expressions are shown on the face prior to or at the beginning of sentences, unless, as happens, then we sense that something is not right or is false. We are aware of timing , although not conscious but we do know. When someone is trying to be too loud or their face is swollen with despair and the tears have drained away or they put their hand down on the table to express frustration, but the gesture was not in sync with what was being spoken, then we can tell there's something wrong.

Make sure you listen

We're more adept at identifying the lies once we hear them and when the pressure is reduced contact.

People are more likely to speak less when they lie. Additionally, people tend to keep the lie in a particular sequence of events, but without providing details. One of the mistakes we make in trying to determine if the person lies is to leap in and claim that we don't believe them.

If you want to know more details about where they werein the moment, what they did specifically and how they felt, then unconscious leakage could happen. Particularly, if you start with the last part of their sequence, and then reverse it in asking them to rectify the sequence of events in case you intentionally misspell something It is possible to find them tangled up in knots. They'll be extremely receptive and irritated by you wanting to know more and extremely defensive, often noting how ridiculous you are for believing in them. "Why would I lie What's the reason?'

If you know someone who typically gives you a lot of details about their experiences and then suddenly displays the most slack or inarticulate manner or just repeats what was practiced so well it is likely they are lying.

They also will distance themselves from the event and will not use the words 'I' or 'Me' in the future. "Oh, sure the usual crowd was there, and the drinks were the same price as they are now'. Then they'll usually follow up by a swift change of topic. In some cases, they will be more detailed and say things like, "Yes that's right, the deal of two for one was over and I was able to have one drink throughout the night!' "Jake was not there, the man said he'd be there, so I'll inquire what he's been doing all night long the next time I meet him. He's a one who lied!' When you feel genuine emotion during the recollection of an event the likelihood is that it's the case.

When you express compliments or polite gestures of gratitude for gifts, such as saying that they are in love with the perfume they received for Christmas , they could mention the way they watched it on television or how costly it was and it's really not a good idea to spend that much, instead of how it smelled and how it affected them personally. This is known as distancing the language. No one would like to lie and the unconscious longs to be honest.

Chapter 13: How to Learn the Six Universal Emotions

When I speak about the body language that is spoken by the face , I'd like to stress the vital distinction between facial body language and different forms that use body language.

The anatomy of the face is distinct due to the fact that the muscles controlling expressions aren't tightly linked to bones. Flexible and loose, they respond to electrical signals emanating from the Lizard brain, which is also known as the limbic brain that was originally developed. In an emergency, a the situation is life or death the lizard brain jumps into action, and takes control and takes control of the whole body. The primitive limbic brain is able to bypass the cerebral cortex that evolved in a much later time and transmits electric signals straight to facial muscles. This is the reason why emotional facial expressions can be uncontrollable, and appear in just a fraction of seconds.

Let's study and understand the various SIX UNIVERSAL expressions of faces:

1. Sadness

2. Surprise

3. Happiness

4. Disgust

5. Anger

6. Fear

SADNESS (SAD FACE)

The most important characteristics of sad expressions on faces expressions include:

1. The outer corners of the eyebrows are lifted and pulled inwards.

2. Simultaneously the lips' corners are pulled down.

How do you judge a sad face?

You'll feel the emotion of sadness when you hold certain expressions.

As in SILENT SUFFERING : This is a kind of suffering that occurs when one is in a position of being alone and is unable to resolve his own issues. You don't need to be silently about the pain you experience or the thoughts that are hurting you.It suggests that you have beginning to look down within your own life.

The different ways a person could be feeling sad or suffer silently of sadness.

#Unhappiness

#Disappointment

#Rejection (might be due to the result of a failure or being rejected by someone)

#Loss

#Sorrow

#Grief

#Mourning

#Despair

#Resignation

All of the above, variations of sadness don't constitute a true kind of sadness.

The true kind of sadness different from the silent kind of suffering as the pure expression of sadness is distinct from the extreme and outward sadness, which is evident through crying, sobbing screaming, or physical manifestations like slapping foreheads or covering the face. Extreme cases begin and then the person is into mild depression.

How can I stop suffering DISEASES?

• Eat healthily, stay clear of sugar and refined food items.

Participate in social activities since this will prevent further isolation.

Get yourself involved in a hectic agenda of working.

Engage in physical activity every day for at minimum thirty minutes per day.

Sadness can deactivate aspects of your Chakra Auric layers and your body and face remain inactive or has started to block slowly. This will not help you to reap the advantages. The cheekbone and eyes begin to dull, and wrinkles start appearing , which are a sign of depression and effects in Kidney.

SURPRISE

It is the second-shortest emotion of all the six Universal emotions.

The Essential Features of Surprise on the face are:

1. Raised eyebrows to the side.

2. Horizontal wrinkles on the forehead.

3. Eyelids are wide open and

4. The Jaws drop - there isn't any tension.

If the person who is astonished by anything, is the first aspect you'll notice on their face is relaxed jaw lines and forehead wrinkles can be the best signs of the surprise. The raised Eyebrows are often misinterpreted as other emotions that can be reflected eyebrows too. Social media is one of the greatest sources of surprises that includes a variety of examples, especially in pranks or video, spontaneous images or more from Facebook, Instagram, WhatsApp etc. That can be a surprise for anyone who sees it shared great memories pictures or memories from the past as well as a video clip of their birthday, anniversary or other celebration.

Chapter 14: What Is It Mean When A Girl or Someone Says "Surprise" Me?

*The phrase "SURPRISE ME " spoken by someone indicates that you are looking for something fresh or different and rid yourself of boredness and make you feel enthused.

How do you make someone surprise and make them smile on their Faces ?

*Plan a day full of fun with lots of little surprises and presents.

*Frame a photograph or an album.

Note or a letter to your beloved ones.

Create a surprise dinner or an event.

You can choose any item that you believe that the recipient will be amazed by your gift.

A person is more joyful because this is a surprise to occur and for most people, it with the spark of a shining Star.It is the time when a the person is healed of minor Issues and Diseases to their daily lives.

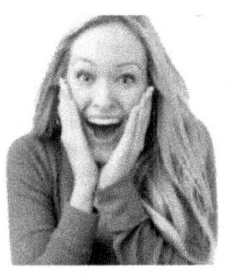

HAPPINESS

It's a completely positive and is the most fundamental Universal facial expressions. Happiness is a feeling everybody wants to be able to experience.

The basic features of happiness that show on your face expressions include:

1. The inside corners of an Eyes pulled in an equal upwards position.

2. The corners of the lips are pulled upwards by an lower jawline.

3. Cheekbone elevated to the side.

The distinction between happiness and pleasure is typically physical, not emotional. You may feel pleasure but not feeling happy. Happiness also distinct from excitement and pleasure since there is a way to be able to enjoy the moment or be overwhelmed without feeling content. Also, remember that the expressions of happiness differ in their intensity.

The most commonly used expression that does not require the use of eyes is a smile for social occasions or another way to say cheese. Check out a politician or Celebrity and you will see that they are all smiling socially in a campaign trial or public gathering.

Happiness is a heightened kind of peace that is within all of us. It makes one feel full active and their Root or Sacral Chakra is active and has positive results in their lives. The negative things slowly disappear from their lives.

Be happy. Keep a smiling face.

DO NOT DISGUISE

"Disgusting" word you use to describe it is offensive, you're expressing your opinion about it for being very unpleasant. Secondly, to declaring something as disgusting is a sign that you think it to be completely unacceptable.

For example :

Like tasting or smelling rotten meat.

Odour of rotten eggs.

Any Peculiar Dirty smell.

A sound of vomiting.

Smoking is a sinful habit...

These, above all, are those that make you make you feel and bring to mind the word "Disgusting".

The Basic Characteristics of a Face with a sexy expression are:

1. The nose is wrinkled.

2. The upper lip is raised as an Snarl.

People often mistake disgust for other emotions. A person might call something offensive, but there is no evidence or even a slight disagreement with something.

Disgusting words make a person unattractive, negative aura and carries all the negative results of

Saturn. People who are disgusted may suffer from skin ailments and have all the negative effects on skin. Wrinkles are likely to appear on their face or body.

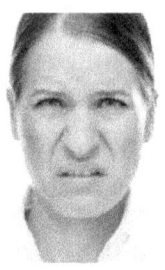

ANGER

"ANGER," as a term, means "Anger" "ANGER" refers to a risky word. emotional state that ranges from anger to out of control Fury.

The basic characteristics of anger in the expression of the face are:

1. Eyebrows are joined.

2 Eyelids are tense.

3. Mouth can be compressed or is open with a square shape.

Anger often appears, when a person is irritated or fatigued, has been experiencing, sustained stress, misbehaved under the influence of alcohol or drugs, unsuccessful into business Ventures, not attaining successful daily life, Short temper, Outbursts of any situation frequently.

Most often, the person was angry because of a myriad of causes of not having a positive mental well-being or even having any thoughts in their head that may trigger an outburst of anger and the person is suffering from this.

Therefore, the most frequent source of anger is a very mentally unstable or troubled thoughts.

As a Face Reader, you have to determine if the person really is mad or is just acting out. In the event that an Expression appears briefly it is likely that he is angered. If the expression is not held when he's angry, then he's acting as if he is angry.

Chapter 15: What Does One Manage Their Anger?

First, by controlling the power of some magical words that suddenly give control to your brain.

Do some exercise and meditation that can help you reduce the risk of anger and instability.

Different facts that affect the body of an individual through anger include:

The body's water level drops and can cause mild dehydration.

The level of blood circulation in the body affects and causes harm to the kidneys, brain, heart and the liver.

The power to make decisions will be diminished or impacted.

The person Kundli the house of lagan is affected.

Sacral Chakra causes bad symptoms or outcomes.

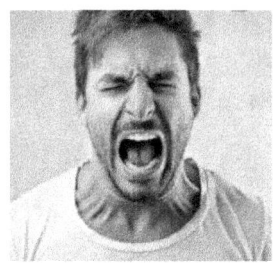

Fear

The most fundamental expression of fear has its roots in the fear of physical or emotional injury The fear has been transformed into a variety of threats , and a man living their life in the fear.

The basic feature of fear on the face expression is:

1. A terrifying face.

2. Eyes are wide-open.

3. Upper lids of the eyes are lifted.

4. Brows can be raised, and pulled together.

5. Mouth open in an oval shape.

The expression that signifies gradation of intensity is due to concern and anxiety, fear anxiety, fearfulness, and stress.

The second reason is that Terror is increased fearfulness that is a fear that is extreme and is a universal and uncontrollable emotion visible in our face. Terror is a type of sudden shock, similar to an intense feeling of anger or a growing worry within your body.

The fear can be reduced through determination and Confidence. Balance your mind by removing the fear that affects you from the inside. You must tackle that anxiety and fight for it instead of being afraid of it.

Insecurity, fear, and anxiety all causes problems for Your Root Chakra, if Root Chakra is affected , then the eye area and temples show darkened skin and dullness. The skin will gradually darker.

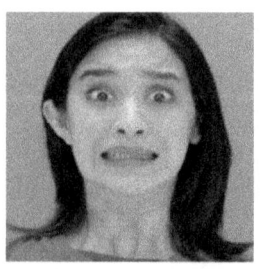

Chapter 16: A Few Combination Face Expressions

The 21 facial expressions are a variety of facial expressions, which are a combination of six Universal expressions such as disgust, anger + sad , etc ..All these expressions help people get over easily from any obstacle or difficulties.

The first expression of face expressions in combination is:

EXPRESSIONS AND BLENDED EMOTIONS:

Blended expressions encompass complex emotions, such as being sad, angry and joyfully in a state of displeasure. This mix of emotions is referred to as COMPOUND EMOTIONS.

The ability to discern facial expressions can add significance and meaning to words. However, blended expressions are a blends of two emotions that leave the person confused about how to proceed or what to avoid doing. If someone is suffering from a mental illness such as Autism asperger,

Asperger or Asperger and also Post Traumatic stress disorder(PTSD) but also you'll have to look at the person who is extremely sensitive to blend of emotions or compounds. In this case, the person is able to be successful with treatments and medications to treat these conditions. You can also look into studying the emotions of people who are and angry, which can be done through the Six Universal emotions.

The SECOND emotion of face expressions in combination is:

LIARS

There are liars everywhere, including innocent people who lie. Little White Lies.

It is a lie that can erode trust and damage us emotionally , often blindly guiding us when we're not prepared.

People are known to lie regularly even when there isn't an evident reason to lie, and even in situations where telling the truth could be more beneficial than telling lies. lie.Those lying with their hands, movements, face expressions, and gestures are quite different from normal.

They are known to smile a lot with their eyebrows raised and their noses are perfectly in a straight
manner. Sometimes, they didn't look into the eyes of someone whom they were telling a lie and didn't make eye contact.

The best way to recognize the truth as an observer is to use your senses without jumping to make a decision .For instance, when you see someone's words conflict with a facial expression, you can tell that something might be wrong.

Now, the THIRD combo of face expression is:

DEAL BREAKER OR MISUNDERSTANDING
Misunderstanding and conflicts can become catastrophic in racially, ethnically,culturally, religiously and economically diverse settings.Think of rabid Sports face, business Rival,Student at rival schools or competing businesses and people with different personalities counter

productive in workplaces where people engage in toxic power games and fail to communicate.

The majority of communications are nonverbal. This is the reason face reading is a crucial skill when you are in an emotionally stressful situation.

Conflicts between words can be devastating when both genders or girls and boys communicate poorly or when someone is rubbing an authority figure the wrong manner.

My personal experience suggests that most couples and families did not have issues due to miscommunication because the primary reason is the fact that they communicate well and aren't afraid to use their words .

In public spaces you could witness a variety of events and frequently see conflict when someone crosses the line, insults someone or invades the space of another. The reason for these conflicts is attitudes, egos and self-respect suffocates the incident. The reason for this is that conflict and miscommunication are caused by a flawed framework of thinking and their mental level. The misperception can be eliminated with the correct and superior understanding.

SEARCH FOR DANGEROUS PEOPLE

Dangerous individuals are of a variety of kinds that is a misguided person, causes tensions between couples because of a misunderstanding, slanders their partner, engages in games of deceit, back biting and the most dangerous are those who take advantage of specific items.

Every one of them have their own motives to make any type of gains and profits in order to fulfil their hopes and goals in the name of jealousy, and certain people simply want the process.

For instance:

"I cannot believe he told me that! I thought he was a good friend".

How can you protect yourself from being a victim of the dangers of the world?

You can determine their credibility by their tricks, or by the motives of the person behind the act.

If anyone you sing with you are more
interested in you, you should look into
the reason behind it and you could be in
issues for you.

A variety of facial expressions reveal
the range of emotions that could
indicate the possibility of danger.

Be aware that facial expressions are
uncontrollable reactions and actions
that speak for themselves .

SOCIAL MASK

The process takes time as well as effort
to discern the difference between our
masks of social identity that are the
faces we show to the world, and the real
feelings and personality attributes.

This is why the majority of us will spend
the rest of our life managing our social
footprints.

We manage our masks for social
occasions depending on what social
conditions demand. If it is we lower our
eyes and purses are lips. We raise our
chins and flesh out our smiles. We
spend the rest of our lives putting on

social identities while protecting our precious life under the shackles.

I've seen many instances where masks for social use are used as essential instruments to protect the privacy of individuals, dignity, and even survival of the mind. Masks are used to disguise and safeguard vulnerable adults and children. "Say cheese! Don't stare! Stand straight! What's wrong to your posture?" I wince when I hear parents disparage the child in public. It's no wonder that adrift teens try on one mask after another in the hope of finding one that makes them famous. Social masks help us establish our identity as well as to communicate with others, and also to measure our abilities. We change this collection of masks through the crucial stages of our lives. We encounter a variety of challenges while we travel through our lives.

I employ THREE methods to get past social masks:

My first method and the most popular method is the close examination of facial expressions-- looking for the exact moment that the person is unconsciously expressing an emotion.

The second method I use -- identifying leaks in the mask requires careful observation. I've seen these leaks in people who use the poker face to conceal their thoughts or feelings. In the same way, a person can't stop the leakage of emotion since the facial expression is without conscious thought.

Third Methodology is

to study and analyse to analyze and observe permanent and fixed expressions, which will be the subject of many of our coming sessions. The physical forms and shapes that are identified as part of Psychological face reading involves observing the way that character traits, emotions as well as attitudes and routine behaviors have formed the physical traits that remain constant to faces.

Is it love at first SIGHT?

There are many reasons why we are compatible and are both attracted to each other. Many couples say that they were in love from the first sight. I'm sure they are right.

A variety of recent psychological studies have shown that mutual attraction is often triggered when we are able to read our faces with precision and sense that the other can sense the emotion we experience in each and every moment. We are most at ease and attracted to those who - we believewe are aware of "where we're to," individuals that "get our feelings," people who are "on our the same page" emotionally etc.

The most fundamental prerequisite for a successful social interaction of lovers is the ability to comprehend motives and feelings of other. To achieve any goal partners need to learn the fundamental skill of analyzing and gathering information regarding the other's behaviour, motives and motives. When we are able to do this then we can collaborate by adjusting our behavior. Individuals who have not yet achieved they have a difficult time working together.

In the field of emotional intelligence,continues to develop

rapidly, but there is general agreement that emotional intelligence involves THREE SKILLS.

Your face-reading training will help you develop yourself.

The most important skill is the awareness of emotionsthe ability to sense and distinguish your own emotions as well as the emotions of other people. The focus was on how you can refine your ability to recognize emotions that others do not see.

The 2nd skill is the practical application of EMOTIONAL intelligence to thinking and, in particular, to resolving PROBLEMS.One of your main jobs is to come up with methods to put the new information you have learned to work. To become a skilled person reader you have to improve your skills by applying your understanding.

The third skill is a powerful managing emotions. This skill blends elements of the previous two abilities. To manage your emotions, you need to be aware of the emotions you experience; to manage your emotions, you have to be able to apply your understanding when you are in emotional situations. Controlling your emotions requires the ability to control your emotions as well as educating yourself to pay attention and affect the moods of others.

Chapter 17: Partition of two Sections Of The Face

This face can be divided in two sections: i.e.

1. Vertically

2. Horizontally

We will now talk the VERTICAL DIVISION OF FACE.

The vertical face division splits the face into two parts i.e. the left and right side that make up the face.

In this case, we split the face in two equally parts starting from the middle of our face, to mid forehead and the chin, as seen in the photo.

The face's vertical division is a place where two high frequencies are present within our bodies that are based on

TWO fundamentals, i.e. SHIV as well as SHAKTI principles.

The right portion of your body controls the Shiva principle while Left side is controlled through the Shakti principle.

The Shiva principle is the male(right) part of our body, and is similar to Yang Energy. Yang Energy is the positive male energy, with all masculine traits and it is Shakti concept is on that of the female(left) part of our body. It is also similar to Yin energy. Yang energy is negative that includes every feminine features.Take into account any religion that you are a part of, they all acknowledge that God has created both women and men to be able to easily adapt to each other because of their nature.

Let's look at what the science tells us. Scientists say that humans mainly use the left side of their brains and the left brain controls the right portion of your body the right-hand part of the physique is considered to be the male one, scientifically speaking, too. Also, regardless of whether you're an right-handed person or left-handed the right side of the body will always be the male/Shiva/Yang part as the other side always remains the female/Shakti/Yin side.

A further fact about left and right sides of the face is that, aside from the fact that it is male is that it also symbolizes the spiritual side. The left side, in addition to being female, represents the physical side of both genders. Shiva side is the supreme Yogi while the other side is the Shakti side is nothing more than the Atma mighta that is the Lord. This is true even when one is talking about the Ardha Nareshwara (half male and half female) divinity Shiva.

Ganpati Ji's truck always points towards the right side for the spiritual worshipers of Ganpati The trucks of Ganpati will be pointed towards the left side of the road for the physical worshippers of Ganpati.

HORIZONTAL DIVISION OF FACE

The face is separated horizontally in three areas, i.e.

1. The Upper Zone

2. Middle Zone, and the Middle Zone, and

3. Lower Zone Lower Zone.

The Horizontal division of the face is divided into three types of material nature.

The upper part of the face is comprised of the upper portion of the forehead, which is located between the eyebrows.

The middle of the face comprises the part between the eyebrows and the nose.

The lower portion of the face comprises the region from the lower part of the nose to the chin.

But, there are times when we find that all three components that make up the face look the same when the person is a mix of all three styles. If any portion or face part is larger than the other parts it is likely that the person is guided by that particular way of life.

Let's discuss the characteristics of the three types of material nature .

1. THE UPPER ZONE OR The CELESTIAL Zone (MODE of Goodness)

If the top part of the face i.e. the forehead is more than the lower and middle areas, then that person is in the good-natured mode. According to the Vedas, people who are in the state of goodness are more pure than other people, since this state of mind is bright and cleanses one of any sinful reaction.

* They work in a mental and an intellectual plane.

They are not afflicted by the plights of material life and are aware of progress in both spiritual and material understanding.

These people are usually poets, writers, philosophers and scientists. They are involved in any area that pertains to the development of mental faculties of an individual.

2. The MIND ZONE (MODE Of PASSION)

The term "belonging" refers to the fact that a person belongs to the category of love in the case that the middle on the face seems larger than the two other parts.

People who are born in this way have unlimited desire and longings . As a result of that, no matter what you do in life, your primary goal is to earn profits as well as the wish to reap the benefits of their efforts.

They also have a body's conception of the world.

They always seek to improve their status, power and their bank balance. If someone is in the pursuit of passion all of their life and passes away in the fashion of love, they take the earth back to live with people who are constantly active and engaged in their material tasks.

The consequences of actions that occur that are performed in the spirit of passion is anxiety, fear, and misery. anxiety.

The people who suffer from this condition tend to be drawn towards an eating plan that is stimulating and can be harsh on the body.

3. THE LOWER ZONE

(MODE of IGNORANCE)

In this instance the lower portion that is on your face has the most long and therefore, these individuals are in a state of ignorance.

They are not engaged like those guided by the concept of desire, and are driven to achieve all things with minimal effort.

Under the influence of ignorance, they are unable to comprehend things properly.

They are not generally at all interested in any sort of spiritual knowledge.

*They would like to sleep from for ten to 12 hours each day, and sometimes even longer and are addicted alcohol.

The people who are in this type of mode tend to be drawn to professions that are based on sexuality or gambling. They are also attracted to intoxicants, gambling and other illegal and unsocial actions. The work done by those who belong to this category is akin to performing without understanding.

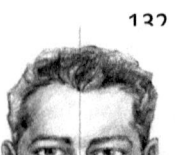

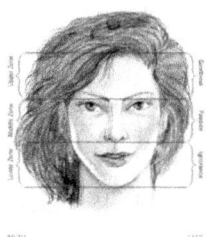

Chapter 18: Eighteen Most Important Facts About Your Face

The first position:

*CENTRAL AXIS on the forehead that indicates the power of Region as well as Divine Consciousness. The central forehead axis is located in the center of forehead. Therefore, if we split the forehead vertically as well as horizontally, and locate the point precisely at the center of the forehead, then it is the central forehead's axis. The central axis of the forehead is an extremely important place of power in the face, and is probably being the one most significant. It is also known as the area of the divine consciousness because it instantly reveals the precise awareness of a person. Beyond spiritual consciousness this area also shows the level of influence a person can have because all ability, authority and control originates from this region.

THE SECOND THE SECOND

The Third Eye Region is often referred to for its role as The Storehouse of Power.It is position just below the central axis that begins at the middle of your eyebrows. This region is a clear indication of the strength of a person or will be in the near future.

The Third Position

The region of the forehead shows that the position begins at the center of the axis and ends at middle of hairline. This is the most prominent area of the forehead and tells how moral and well-informed a person. The forehead region reveals how impartial and patient the person has, how the amount of faith, belief and trust a person has, and whether or not the person is a believer in integrity, honesty and loyalty.

THE 4TH Position

The REGIONS OF FAME and wealth, as well as enjoyment. This area is situated between the eyebrows. The Right eyebrows is related to glory, effulgence, magnificence, illustriousness, noble things, fame, or power a person will have in his life and how noble spirited a person is. Also, the left Eyebrows are a source of the appearance of pleasure, beauty and sex, as well as luxurious, wealth and also tells how much a person can take pleasure from the results of his work in his life . It also tells what sort of life and what kind of pleasures the person can expect to have in his lifetime and whether the person is going to enjoy some enjoyment and pleasure or need to work hard all through his life.

THE FIFTH Position

THE TRANSITION POINT BETWEEN MODE of GOODNESS and MODE of PASSION indicates that this is an extremely significant area, as it is the place where you begin the bridge of the nose and also as the transition point between the good side towards the state of love. This area is responsible for ensuring a balanced flow of energy between the two areas. Therefore, the skin of this region should be soft and clean. The structure of this region is crucial because this region provides details on the way a person utilizes his or her knowledge and abilities to success in achieving various items such as wealth and fortune.

THE SIXTH POSITION

The physical, mental, and financial structure of a PERSON The bridge of the NOSE. This indicates that the bridges of the nose are crucial in determining the general health and constitution of an individual. When the bridge on the nasal is weak and unlucky it will influence the health of the person and that person will have an unsound physical constitution.

The seventh position:

The CHARACTER and WEALTH of the tip of the nose indicates that the nose's tip is the primary factor in character and wealth. A beautiful nose is one that is crystal smooth, clear and free of markings or cracks.

THE EIGHTH POSITION

The fact that the EYES HAVE an inner power that is able to bring about HEALTH and vitality. HONESTY and Intelligence. that the eyes have the greatest importance within the body. Eyes are such an essential asset that, if they hadn't been around, we would not be able to see or appreciate the beauty of the world, and everything would've been dark. The eyes are among the primary element that determines the various aspects of an individual's behavior and personality.

THE TENTH POSITION

The region directly beneath the EYES is often referred to as family relationships. This is crucial when it comes to revealing information concerning a person's relations with their family members. If under the eye, there's a concern that's revealed conflicts within the family and discord.

THE NINTH POSITION

The EYEBROWS as well as the area between the EYELIDS and the EYEBROWS shows the personal relationship between parents and SIBLINGS. This region is a an important position on the face since it shows a healthy relationship between siblings and parents. If there is any wrinkles or dullness or any other problems arise in this region that indicates conflict and tension within their relationships.

THE TWELFTH POSITION

The CHEEKS AND THE CHEEKBONES demonstrate the dominance and aggression.

The cheeks and cheekbones are crucial in determining the personality of a person's character in terms of aggression, dominance and authority.If an area of concern is this , it will show an aggressive behavior, dominating persona and governing everyone around them. This can cause stress and discomfort within their lives.

THE ELEVENTH POSITION

The CORNERS OF YHE EYES is referred to as FOR Sexual Relationships.

The eyes' corners are the most important indicator of a person's sexuality and the position is given to lover, wife and loved ones. It is an extremely important facial area when a person's sexuality is to be evaluated.

THE THIRTEENTH POSITION

The ears are of WISDOM and FORTUNE

The ears are among the most vital part of the face, eyes assist us see the world, just as the ears aid us in our ability to understand and listen to the world around us. The ears are also crucial in reading faces because the ears assist us in determining the wisdom and the fortune of an individual.

THE FOURTEENTH THE FOURTEENTH

*THE PHILTRUM showcases the hottest sexual appetite.

The philtrum plays a crucial facial area and can reveal the sexual desire of the person. It also informs us about procreation and productivity and the physical structure of an individual.

THE SIXTEENTH POSITION

REGION OF FA LINGLINES that is also commonly referred to as REGION of ADMINISTRATIVE Skills.

This is a way to determine the level of administrative ability of a person as well as what they know about them and have higher professional capabilities.

THE FIFTY-TEENTH THE POSITION

THE MOUTH shows MINDSET, PERSONALITY, NATURE, SENSUALITY, APPETITE, WEALTH, etc.ETC.

The mouth is considered to be an extremely vital places on the face. The mouth assists us in figuring out a variety of aspects about an individual, as the mouth is a representation of our profession and business, as well as appetizers attraction, appearance, controlling strength, intelligence, and wealth .

THE SEVENTEENTH POSITION

THE CHIN shows LEADERSHIP QUALITIES .

The chin is specifically concerned with leadership skills as well as rules and discipline, and the ability to deal with any situations. If there is any issue on your chin, it can cause problems in the these qualities of a person.

THE EIGHTEENTH POSITION

Travel and MOVEMENT is indicated by the SIDES OF FOREHEAD. This is just below the CORNERS of the eyebrows.

These positions are important to spot in our lives because they aid in determining if a person is lucky enough to be traveling. These positions also tell whether traveling will be beneficial or result in loss. The more clear and shiny skin indicates the number of opportunities for travel and international career or business activities.

Chapter 19: Category The Face In Its Width

BROAD FACE:

Wide faces tend to be bigger than normal facial features. The foreheads of these faces are usually wider.

The faces could also be alike in dimensions, giving a an appearance of squarish face. These individuals are typically more liberal and open-minded than most people.

The judgments and decisions they make are largely influenced by logic and knowledge. Due to their high tolerance levels they are able to withstand external influences with ease, without difficulty.

They also possess good ability to influence others as they're usually not affected by external influences like temperatures, politics or bad behavior, and their decision-making process tends to be controlled by their confidence, faith and confidence in their own authority.

Someone with a broad face is also confident. The combination of these traits with a broad-minded view make them excellent managers.

This is why you'll be able to see that the majority of managers around the globe have wide faces.

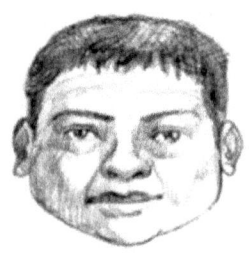

NARROW FACE

A thin face can be seen because it appears appear thinner than normal. A narrow face is higher that its wide. The width of face tends to narrow.

But don't be confused between thin and oblong-faced faces, since most oblong faces are wide with wide foreheads.

People with a narrow facial profile typically have foreheads that are narrow too, but you won't see all of them with small foreheads. People with narrow foreheads have a restricted perspective on the world. They have little or any tolerance for others particularly when things don't always go in their way.

The reason for this is that they are extremely impatient, and can become extremely stressed, angry or even angry when any pressure is put on them. Due to this, they can sometimes exaggerate even small things out of the realm of possibility.

They have no tolerance and do not feel fully satisfied with anything. They expect more from others and situations. Someone with a narrow-minded view may be extremely confident from experiences, but not by nature.

It means that when they are trying something new, one might be anxious or afraid.

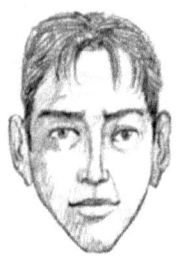

Face age area

AGES 1-14:

The ages of one to fourteen are on the ear. Therefore, the success of a person's years is reflected in the ears.

Ages 1 to 7 are ordered in a sequential order from top to the bottom on the left EAR as well as the ages of eight to fourteen are in the same manner on the right EAR.

In determining the quality of life for individuals aged between one and fourteen years old, the growth of ears needs to be assessed with care. If ears are deformed and are not functioning properly, the child will be born into a family in which they are not cared for well by parents at the ages of. It is likely that the parents won't be financially secure. When the size of an ear appears small, in most instances it means that the first year until the age of 14 will be a tumultuous time for the child. However, smaller ears do not mean that the child will be lacking financial resources throughout their lives. The person could become richor poor determined by the actions he/she takes and the advice and guidance that they receive throughout their lives.

AGES 15-30:

The age group 15-30 is found within the region over the eyes, i.e. your entire forehead.

Fifteen begins at the middle of the forehead. It then from 16 onwards, it drops and covers the entire forehead. Age 28 is found on the 3rd area, located in the middle of both brows. the ages of 29 and 30 are in the left and right temples, respectively.

A poorly-formed forehead can indicate poor memory, insufficient intelligence, and many other obstacles in this age.

AGES 35-43:

The AGE-GROUP 35-43 is depicted by EYES as well as the AREA the EYES.

The eye and space surrounding them must be clean and bright in order to be considered to be in the auspicious category.

If however, there are dark spots or crisscross designs, those who suffer from them carry a huge burden and are often unhappy. If the eye region is not in a good place, they will be suffering a lot. A few of them could be punished by the courts for certain crimes. This type of lawful entrapment generally occurs between 35-42.

AGES 51-73:

It is believed that the AGE 51 is represented by the PHILTRUM.

The AGE-GROUP 52-5 is represented by the upper part of the LIPS.

AGES 56,57 64, 65, 68 as well as 69, are represented in the FA LING LING.

The AGE GROUPS they are able to see that the Fa Ling lines have a significant impact on the ages of 55 and 57.

SIXTY represents SIXTY is represented by MOUTH, i.e. the LIPS. Likewise, the AGE-GROUP between 61 and 63 and 66-67, are represented by the PORTION ABOVE the LIPS.

Age-GROUP 70-73 is represented in THE CHIN. The health of people in this age group will be largely dependent on the significance and unluckiness of the position of these characteristics on the face.

The majority of people die during this time. It is usually due to defective Fa Ling lines, mouths and the chins.

AGES 44-50:

Ages 41, 44, and 45 are represented in the bridge of the nose.

Ages 47 and 46 are represented in CHEEKS and the CHEEKBONES.

The AGE-GROUP 48 is represented with the tip of the nose The AGES 49 and 50 can be represented with the NOSE'S WINGS.

If there are dark spots on the nasal bridge, or on the cheeks or cheekbones, the person may have serious health issues particularly between the ages of 41-47.

Dark patches, scars etc. may also trigger drastic alteration of relationships. In the event that the nose seems not straight or is damaged that indicate an untrue character as well as financial limitations.

The people who suffer from this condition may experience quite a bit during AGES 45-50.

AGES 75-100:

The ages are determined from the SIDE OF THE CHIN that go around the CIRCUMFERENCE OF FACE, circling across the face, making a complete circle, before coming back down the chin to complete the complete cycle of 100 years.

In general, people don't reach the age of seventy-nine.

If a person is in the age of seventy, and especially the seventy-fifth year, it's time to reflect for the person.

If we examine the circles the AGES (74-100) create and observe the circle, we can see that it's in the clockwise direction. This means that if one needs to find major events or events in the age range, they must create an equivalence of different ages. It is important to remember that everything that happens in the universe happens in a coordinated and synchronized manner...

Important Note:

As you calculate however, it is considered both right side (of the face as well as the body) are different for females and males.

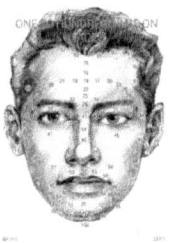

This is the moment to begin A SERIES of FASHIONABLE Features of OUR Face-to-face one-on-one.

Here, we begin with OUR first FEATURE ....

(HAIR)

FACIAL SECRETS

HAIR

Venus is the ruler of hairs. As one of the many aspects of one's personality, hair can reflect the temperament, sexual preferences as well as other idea-related details. The various types and styles of hair also have a connection to one's ethnicity, race and the region where they were born.

Hair colour varies dimensions, size, and shape for every person. The individual hair's colours are different due to the melanin that is that is present and also according to differences in the surface shape and distribution of the hair. Hair quality is a factor that determines the form of hair.

If, for instance, hair is rough or kinky, then it will be cut into ribbons that resemble twisted.

DIFFERENT types of hair

1. Fine, smooth and straight HAIR

a. Hair that is silky soft and silky indicates it is a sign that Yang forces within are in control.

b. They exhibit controlled behavior and, even when they are extremely angry, they will not reveal their anger to other people.

C. They possess a good quantity of fire element in their bodies. They don't suffer from stomach-related issues.

2. Dry, rough and coarse HAIR

a. Hairy people who are dry, rough and coarse are flooded with Yang inside their hair.

b. The fire element isn't in control, which is why these individuals suffer from stomach issues.

C. They are extremely argumentative and are known to argue over every little detail. If they have dry lips, then they are prone to wicked behavior too.

D. They often suffer the most throughout their lives.

3. CURLY HAIR

a. Women who have high levels of oestrogen and those who have high testosterone levels are likely to be curly.

b. Hairy people are sexually attractive and possess massive sexual appetites. People with curly hair are also used to activities of leisure.

C. Hairy children tend to be more interested in activities outdoors So don't be shocked to observe them growing to become world-renowned players in one sport.

4. SCATTERED HAIR

a. Don't confuse this with messy and hair that isn't combed. It's a term used to describe the hair growing in various directions.

b. Therefore, this hair doesn't develop in a sequential way.

C. Hair-loss sufferers are prone to having a tense mind and are unable to concentrate their attention to a specific objective or goal.

5. BALDING

a. The early balding that occurs before reaching the age 45 is a sign of the person's weakening body.

b. These individuals are extremely attracted to, interested in and obsessed with sexual issues.

C. Thus the strong sex drive of these women is a important reason for the baldness. Another reason for their early baldness is tendency to be impulsive.

D. People who are quickly angry and the frenzies of anger occasionally can cause the appearance of baldness.

It is a. But, it must be noted that if individuals get bald at the age of 50 it is a sign of the growth of a spiritual mind.

CATEGORISATION OF HAIR IN ACCORDANCE to its thickness

1. Thick HAIR

a. Hair that is dense and strong suggests that the individual has a an extremely robust physical constitution.

They are mostly emotional creatures.

b. They may also be aggressive, inflexible and over-reactive.

2. Thin and delicate hair

a. Hair that is fragile and thin hair don't have a lot of endurance , and they are physically fragile.

b. People with these types of build tend to have a higher risk of being fragile when their body is thin.

3. even THICKNESS/NORMAL AIR

a. Normal hair is one that is not too thin or too thick. It's not too dense or brittle, and neither is it very thin, fragile and delicate.

b. Hairs with equal thickness have well-balanced personalities.

C. They also have artistic talent and are aware of their environment and behavior.

CATEGORISATION OF HAIR ACCORDING to its length

1. LONG HAIR

Vedic texts declare that Kama lives in hair, and the longer the hair grows, more intense are the flutters of love.

Hair with long hair is also believed to be a symbol of modesty, royalty as well as wealth and pleasure.

The Vedas tell us that women who have lengthy hair can be blessed by virtue luck, chastity and fame.

Princes, warriors, and monarchs wore long hair in the ancient times of India because it was believed to be a mark of royalty.

2. SHORT HAIR

Short haired people tend to be impulsive. The fashion of wearing short hair first emerged around the West and spread throughout Asia.

The rulers and warriors of the Roman Empire are depicted with long hair. The first mention of shorter hair came from the depiction in the portrayal of Normans along with those of the Knights from the West probably in the 11-12th century.

The Knights who embarked on long expeditions would cut their hair extremely short, since it was believed to indicate roughness.

Hair Types and Categories based on different colours and textures.

1. BLACK HAIR

Hairy people who have BLACK hair naturally have more MELANIN inside their hair than blonde counterparts. It is crucial to recognize that melanin an HORMONE produced in the PINEAL GLANDS within the body. They are produced by cells known as MELANOCYTES.

There are MULTIPLE benefits of MELANIN It is for instance that melanin functions as a mechanism for taking in sun's heat blocking UV rays, protects the skin from cancer, and is an anti-aging hormone that helps prevent wrinkles as well as the other symptoms of ageing. The melanin concentration within your body can be the primary element that determines the appearance of an individual. It is named a mental and PHYSICALLY STIMULATING hormone.

People who have black hair certainly contain higher levels of hormone stimulants than those who have blonde hair. Melanin isn't only responsible for the color of hair. It also influences for the appearance, as well as the color of eyes.

Therefore, those with white skin, light hair color and eyes with light-coloured shades are genetically deficient since they have hormonal issues. People who are very white, have low melaninlevels, and also suffer from freckles, indications of aging rapidly wrinkles wrinkles, and cancer, etc.

6. NARROW at the top of the forehead

This type of forehead has a an angular appearance and a thick hair growth along the side. They are blocked in their professional and personal life. They don't have the ability to realize their goals. There is a barrier in their socio-economic values, or maintaining positive relationships. Keep your teeth clean for a better analysis. The use of perfume is mandatory. Always keep a white hankerchief on your purse at all times.

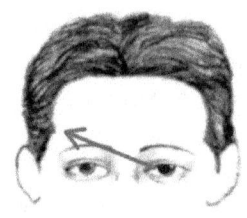

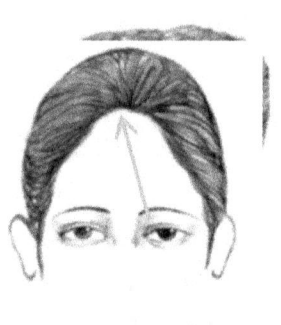

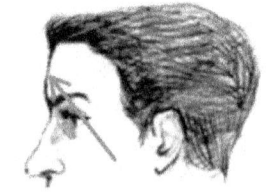

7. SHALLOW FOREHEAD

A slender forehead and an unnatural hairline indicates problems in their professional life. It could also be a sign of trouble with parents between 15 and 30 years old. They generally be extremely hardworking and can make a name for themselves when they reach 30.Don't achieve immediately if they are in search of jobs.Do workship at the Tulsi plant and water it regularly. Chant Gayatri Mantra daily.

8. PROTRUDING FOREHEAD

Forheads that are protruding from the sides are usually asymmetrical and curved at the front, creating the appearance of a convex forehead. A person is a an avid dreamer. They should be able to hold their thoughts slowly before working toward achieving it. They aren't rushing to grasp something new before making decisions.Their professional and personal lives require a balanced approach to ensure they are running well. People who take their time or think twice before starting a new startup.Be honest and have a realistic attitude towards life.Clean your teeth and your nose Every day for betterment in your life.

Disease

[15:13 29/10/2020] Research by Prateekvastu Ins: Dentification of diseases through face reading . To detect various diseases by reading faces one must be acquainted in the

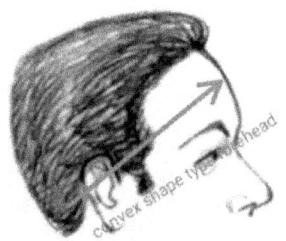

facial regions that control the inner organs of the body. The following are the ones:

(1) The topmost portion of the skull controlled by the kidneys.

(2) 2. The foreground symbolises the bladder.

(3) The region above the eyebrows is controlled by the gall bladder.

(4) The space between the brows is controlled by the liver and stomach.

(5) Thyroid organs, kidneys, and liver are symbolized by the eyebrows

(6) The eye's under area is the stomach, kidneys and the liver

(7) The nose and cheeks represent the heart region.

(8) 8. The upper portion of the cheeks as well as jaws are a representation of the stomach, lungs, and colon

(9) The sides of the nose are the lung.

(10) 10. The ears are the kidney.

(11) (11) The philtrum symbolizes the area of the spleen.

(12) The area that is above the upper lip refers to the liver.

(13) (13) The stomach symbolizes the upper lip.

(14) 14. The stomach is the lower lip.

(15) The regions between the mouth's apex are symbolized by the colon

(16) 16) The chin controlled by the bladder and kidneys.

1. Vertical lines above the end of the eyebrows. the position on the forehead determined by gall bladder the presence of vertical lines that appear in this area or any other area of the forehead indicate some issues or strain on the gall bladder. Lines with cross-hatched or spots on the forehead can also signify obstruction of the kidneys and gallbladder. This could be caused by excessive oily and oily food items, or the excessive consumption of alcohol and cigarettes. A lot of stress on the gall-bladder and liver could cause headaches, dizziness and more.

2. Lines of cross-hatching between the eyebrows: These lines are a sign of serious problems within the stomach or liver. Most often, these individuals have a problem with alcohol due to continuous internal conflict and imbalance that could cause liver damage.

3. Unsuspecting marks that are located on the forehead These can cause hypertension and liver complications and kidneys, as well as dizziness.

4. Dark brows begin to fade at the middle can indicate thyroid issues.

5. Blue veins appear on the cornea If the cornea turns blue or blue veins are visible on the cornea, this suggests a issue in the liver or kidney. It could also be a sign of depleting adrenal energy.

6. The cornea is covered with yellow veins The presence of yellow veins on the cornea indicates an issue with the kidneys, liver or both. The presence of permanent blue or yellow veins on the cornea could indicate an issue with the kidneys or liver. kidneys of a person could be permanently damaged.

7. Darkness, puffiness or cross-hatched lines under the eye area This signify an abundance of internal strife and disturbance inside a person. A majority of them suffer from addiction to alcohol, drugs as well as other intoxicants. If you notice an increase in puffiness or crossed-hatched lines, this could be a sign of problems in the liver, stomach or

kidneys. In some instances, it may indicate liver damage, particularly when moles or other suspicious signs are visible within this area. Darkening and puffiness under the eyes can also indicate adrenal depletion due to excessive sleep, worry drinking or worrying about junk food.

8. The lines that run across the cheeks and from the corners of the eyes could indicate a issue with the kidneys or in the intestine.

9. Ear redness The cause of ear redness suggests that the kidney or liver is under strain because of unhealthy food, drinks, or smoking cigarettes. The redness of the ear also suggests the loss of the adrenal gland's energy.

The mouth and the lips symbolize the stomach as well as the parts of the intestines. The part over the upper lip is the liver. It is depicted in the lower region of the face, as well as the jaws. If a person is suffering from constipation or any other stomach related issues, pimples and boils are visible on the lips and in other areas that comprise the facial area. A diet-related disorder, excessive in sugar, dairy and junk food may cause mouth soreness as well as cracked lips. pimples or white spots on the lower part of your face. Blotchy and white spots could also indicate yeast infections. If your lips appear dry or cracked it could be a sign of acidity and inside heat in the stomach. Lips that protrude out indicate an unresponsive colon. Dryness in the mouth is a sign of the presence of heat in the stomach.

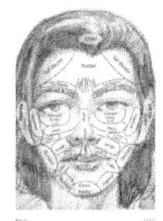

LIPS

LIPS denotes our planet Mars. Lips are composed of lower lips which is mars's bad side and the upper lip, that are good mars. Lips are a way to determine how attractive a person is. LIPS influence a person's sexual desires and are a major indicator of how kind or selfish someone is. Since the eyes are the windows to the soul, so the lips can be a entrance to the person's personality and personality. Let's gauge our sexual appetite and our capacity to woo others in the context of a romantic relationship. In the face reading the mouth and lips indicates how much luck the person will experience by the time they reach 60. Lips are the most important indicators of financial health. Therefore, the lips must be thoroughly assessed and observed.

The various types of lips are as follows:

1. Full LIPS or THICK LIPS

Lips with a thick lip are usually very sensual and devoted to pleasure. They are awed by food and are fervent eaters.They also possess a beautiful nature. Lips that are full of aplomb can be a sign of the warmth of a personality.Lips are full of a sense of the degree to which Frank or open the person. It's all about the self disclosure.Thick lips are ideal for women, but not for men. It is common for women who strip in fashion magazine or carry out the same work, have full lips. Full lips indicate that the person is content with their own persona, however if they lift an extremely thicklip indicates an exaggeration of the person's behavior, attitude and appearance. The character and behavior are most likely to be uncertain. Make sure to use silver and make use of the maximum amount of silver ornaments, tools, etc.

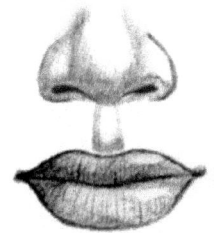

2. POUTING LIPS

Pouting lips are designed with by thick lips, with the ends facing towards the upwards. The sexual desire of these individuals is extremely robust. They are also in need of the love and affection of others and need continuous nourishment throughout their early years and also. Lips are also a sign of good health, financial the ability to make friends for a long time .Pounting lips also indicates the presence of a

An unresolved emotional streak within the character. They are also very unpredictable with a continuous change in mood. If their lips aren't the only feature of their face are attractive and attractive, then they'll have great financial reserves .Avoid all triangles .Do the work of a female goddess. A silver ring should be worn on your finger.

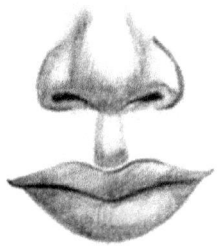

3. Thin LIPS

People with thin lips are extremely preoccupied. Lips that are thin also signify an extremely dominating and control personality. They want to be in total authority over all things. If their lips are thin and broad, they are the type who control all around them and are very powerful. Because of their dominant controlling and cautious nature , they are not a fan of speaking about their life or teaching them things. They're not generous, are extremely calculating and usually have a self-centered attitude. Beware of too many events and celebrations. Silver is essential to ease your daily problems. Beware of eating food before bedtime.

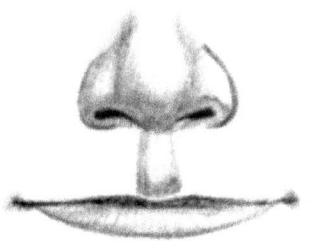

4. MODERATE LIPS WITH THICKNESS

The lips of this type that are not too thick or thin is thought to be the finest out of everyone. The people with these lips have an even temperament, a fine and flexible character. They don't talk too much or in a way that isn't useful. They are family-oriented and help their family members. They do not display excess zeal in eating, sleeping, or any other things and are extremely well-balanced. Keep a square piece of silver in your bag. Beware of any triangles that are surrounding you.

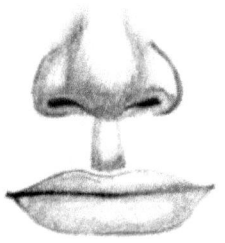

5. OVAL LIPS

Oval lips are round corners. Some people are slow to take decisions but once they've taken an important decision, they are unthinking and quickly execute their decision. They are extremely sensual. They tend to be insane and confused people. They have a good sense of finances and have luxury lodging. They can achieve their goals through methods. Being patient and a commitment to nature. Have an excellent personality and character. Avoid eating food at night. Make use of silver utensils, or jewelry for yourself, or do not give silver for gifts to anyone.

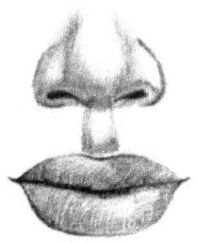

6. LIPS DISTRATED OR CROOKED

These kinds of people aren't fair nor are they truly honest. They have a few grey hues. People with a crooked mouth have unbalanced thoughts and a poor character. They are prone to cheating and are very impatient the way they behave. You can tell lies about all things. Being in financial and personal trouble. Avoid excessive Celebration. A nasturtious salted namkeen is served as an Prasad on a Tuesday or a Saturday in the hanumanji temple.

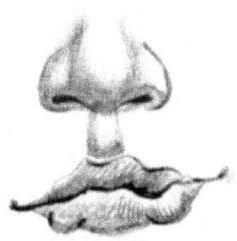

CHIN

Chin is our kundali 2nd house. Chin denotes Mars planet. Chin plays a significant role as a support for your lower facial. Chin predicts leadership qualities, strength character, and will.It must be remembered that the chin is a source of dominance and can predict a person's whether they are strong-hearted or weak-hearted. is easily determined by looking at the cheeks. Chin indicate what people's lives will look in the seventies.

These types of chains are:

1. POINTED CHIN

A chin that is pointed are triangular in shape. People with a pointed Chin are not content to be alone as they are in a constant need to connect with others and draw attention to everyone. They are controlled by emotions , and may not be content with one thing or relationship.They are susceptible to mood swings in short intervals.These people can also be anxious and make rapid decisions. Keep your temper in check and don't be involved in arguments. Be patient in your handling of the marriage will yield positive results.Try to stay clear of red clothing. Keep or wear silver along with you.

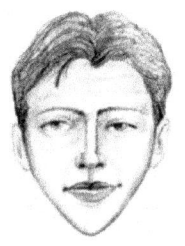

2. SQUARE CHIN

Square Chin have a squarish outline. People who have square Chin are extremely demanding when it comes to love as well as personal relations. They lack humour and possess a tough personality. The square chin can also show stubbornness. It's difficult for people with a squarish chin to recognize their own shortcomings or shortcomings. They have a tendency of seeing faults in others. They can also be Moody and impatient. They don't want to be patient for a long period of time, and if their patient is being tested, they may become violent and violent. Recite Hanuman Chalisa regularly and Gayatri Mantra 108 times during the day. Donating blood helps lessen the effects of this type of nose.

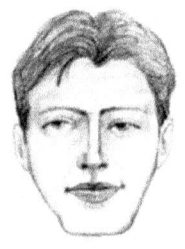

3. ROUND CHIN

People who have round chins are kind, courteous and family-oriented. They are also adept at listening and giving tips. They are able to maintain their relationships well and are successful at every level in their lives. Then, recite Hanuman Challisa or Gayatri Mantra at least 108 times throughout the day. Do not wear or use red color. Give out sweets at the vicinity of a temple or other holy places.

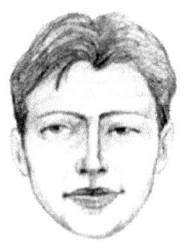

4. FLESHY CHIN

The chins that are fleshy contain a padded tissues within the chin. These individuals have an unpleasant style of working and are not extremely tolerant or even moderate. If they also have a an overly large or protruding jaw, as well as prominent cheekbones or cheeks and cheekbones, they'll be tyrants , like Saddam Hussein. They can be extremely violent, aggressive and abusive. They are prone to taking revenge.Have the ability to manage the anger and abuse. Use a the red napkin or handkerchief in your purse. Recite Hanuman Chalisa. Be honest and maintain morality.

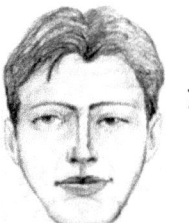

5. Turned up CHIN

If the point of Chin is raised to form an horizontal line or cut in the chin area, those who have a chin cleft are stubborn and display the same characteristics and traits like those who have a fleshy cheeks. Being rude and harsh. Must work hard and be a slave in their life. Take a small piece of silver along with you. Feeding monkeys is another method of tranquil Mars. Avoid wearing or using Red color.

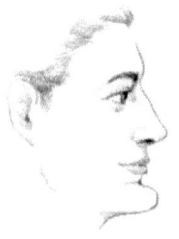

6. CHIN RERECEDING

The chins that receding are angled inward toward the throat. This is the exact opposite behavior and characteristics. They lack confidence and tend to be scared easily by any type of contest. They are afraid to speak in public with other people of the same gender. They require lots of buttering and praise. The main issue for them is to overcome be able to cope with the pressure of an unneeded adulteration as well as to overcome their childlike attitude and behavior more maturely. Be in control of your anger by doing meditation. Bring sweets to the temple or a religious spot. Don't lie or deceive anyone and maintain an ethical character.

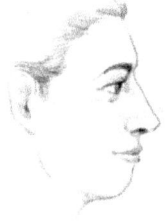

Teeth

Teeth is the third house of the kundli. Teeth denotes Mercury planet. Teeth play an important part in the face reading. The way that teeth are set is an essential factor in determining the temperament and character of an individual. A healthy smile can provide a positive performance in both career and business. A poor dental health can create obstacles and challenges to your professional and personal life.

The various kinds of teeth are:

1. TETH WITH NO GAPS INSIDE THEM

If there aren't any gaps between two teeth, and the teeth are tightly packed with each other on both sides, then that is the best position for the teeth. They are also observant and have even temperaments. They are also generous and usually care about of the other's wants and needs and needs. They don't make a the decision-making process quickly. They are sensible, deliberate and methodical in their decisions. Make sure you clean your teeth regularly. Use mouth freshener or Sauf for healthy teeth. If there is any deformity or defect in your teeth, consult a dentist for treatment the problem as soon as you can for the best astrological benefits.

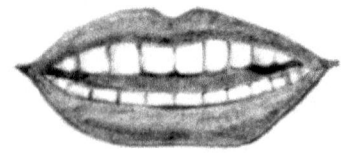

2. Uneven Teeth

Uneven teeth are usually experienced by people who have no temperaments and are extremely unstable. They also have in the same way as those with mean, sloppy and unreliable characteristics. They typically exhibit wicked behavior in the event of gaps in between their teeth .These teeth signify the presence of animal-like behavior because If you only look at their teeth on any animal, you will be amazed to find that they all have teeth that are uneven. They also signify uneven life and heavy load throughout their lives. Take Fitkari daily water gargles at night to minimize the effects of these kinds teeth. teeth.Use to drink Sauf and Mishri following meals.

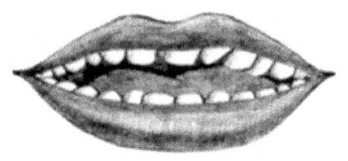

3. SPACED Teeth

The teeth with gaps are spaced between them.Same as mentioned above, these teeth are also characterized by animal-like behavior. They have a base character and are very unselfish, mean, mean as well as abrasive and
veil. They're among those who are purely focused on their own needs and don't pay attention to moral
values. Take Fitkari water gargles, which reduce the effects of these kinds of teeth. Take a bite of sauf and Mishri immediately after eating.

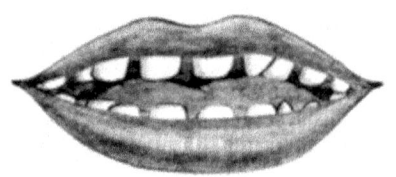

4. SPACED FRONT TETH

If there's a gap between the front and back teeth, which are located between the upper and lower front two teeth it is a sign of the most foolish and cheap nature people.There is always a miracle on them, and they receive their possessions on time, when they need to. They enjoy taking risks , and often expressions of anger and outrage at people's faces. After dinner, make sure to drink regular water. Consume more green vegetables and chutneys with greens into your meals.

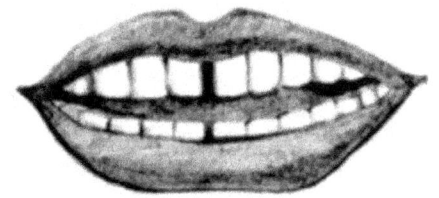

Conclusion

By combining this knowledge together with your own practice skills and knowledge, you will not only be a better practitioner, but also gain the skills to detect diseases or illnesses within the body by looking at the appearance. The problem is that courses and books focus too much on theoretical details. We read faces of people every day , but we don't know the content we read.

If we can begin to comprehend the content we are reading and absorbing the information, it can help our study and observations. Faces can be changed by pursuing a healthy way of life. The changes that appear on their faces indicate that the organs are in good shape.

www.ingramcontent.com/pod-product-compliance
Lightning Source LLC
Chambersburg PA
CBHW050403120526
44590CB00015B/1802